Here's How to Do Stuttering Therapy

Here's How Series

Thomas Murry, PhD
Series Editor

Here's How to Treat Childhood Apraxia of Speech by Margaret A. Fish

Here's How Children Learn Speech and Language: A Text on Different Learning Strategies by Margo Kinzer Courter

Here's How to Do Stuttering Therapy by Gary J. Rentschler

Here's How to Do Stuttering Therapy

Gary J. Rentschler, PhD

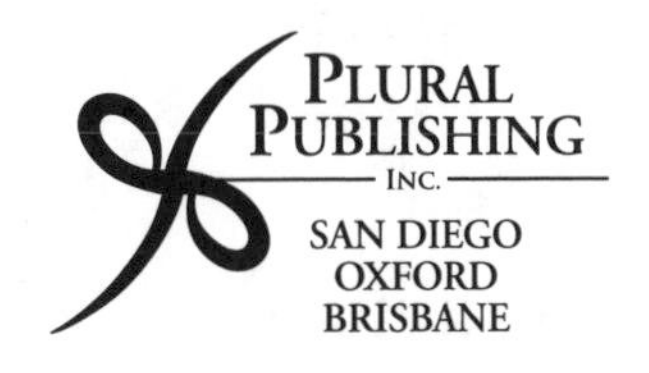

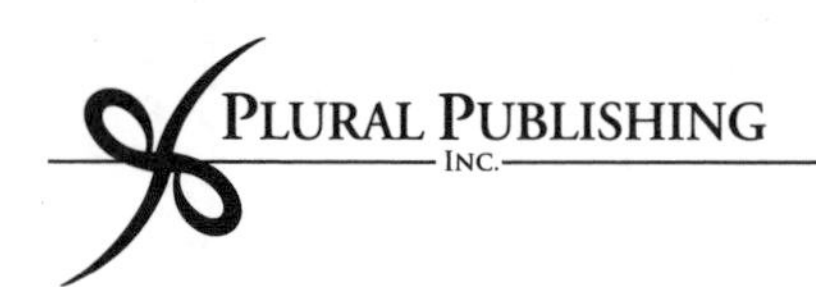

5521 Ruffin Road
San Diego, CA 92123

e-mail: info@pluralpublishing.com
Web site: http://www.pluralpublishing.com

49 Bath Street
Abingdon, Oxfordshire OX14 1EA
United Kingdom

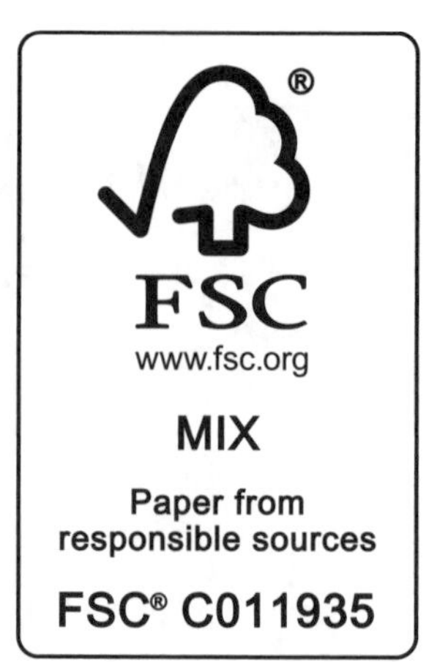

Typeset in 11/15 Stone Informal by Flanagan's Publishing Services, Inc.
Printed in the United States of America by McNaughton and Gunn

Library of Congress Cataloging-in-Publication Data

Rentschler, Gary J., 1947-
Here's how to do stuttering therapy / Gary J. Rentschler.
p. ; cm. — (Here's how series)
Includes bibliographical references and index.
ISBN-13: 978-1-59756-386-4 (alk. paper)
ISBN-10: 1-59756-386-2 (alk. paper)
1. Stuttering--Treatment. 2. Counseling. I. Title. II. Series: Here's how series.
[DNLM: 1. Stuttering--therapy. 2. Counseling--methods. 3. Speech Therapy—methods. WM 475.7]
RC424.R46 2011
616.85'54--dc23

2011022080

Contents

Foreword

The "Here's How Series" is a collection of texts that go directly to a "hands on" approach to understanding and treating a specific disorder. This series emanated out of an observation that speech-language pathologists who work in varied environments, hospitals, clinics, school systems, and private practice were buyers of the book, *Here's How to Do Therapy* by Debra Dwight. Debra's unique "here's how" approach was intended primarily for young clinicians. However, records show that not only young clinicians but also experienced clinicians, teachers, and students were also buying the book. Soon after the purchase of that book, however, clinicians were asking for a similar book but with more detail about specific topics—child language, autism, fluency, and literacy, to name a few. This series offers exactly that, an in-depth approach to specific topics.

Each author in the "Here's How Series" is a clinician first and foremost in his or her area of speech-language pathology. Each brings years of experience with success to support that experience. You won't find extensive reference lists but you will find the author's well-documented and success driven practices to the topics discussed. You, the clinician, will find practical information to raise your clinical practice to the next higher level. And, you'll enjoy sharing the author's experiences through the pages brought to life with case studies, case vignettes, and clinical tips based on the author's experiences. We hope you enjoy Plural Publishing's "Here's How Series."

Dr. Rentschler's approach to stuttering therapy breaks down the challenges of treating children as well as adults by offering lesson plans, treatment modules, and activities appropriate to both the child and adult who stutter. His section on activities includes approaches to managing anxiety, overcoming shame, and how to deal with avoidance of stuttering situations. The clinician will appreciate the sections on resources and support that he has gathered to aid the clinical process.

Thomas Murry, PhD
Series Editor

Preface

Throughout this book the distinction is made between childhood and adult experiences with stuttering. The difference is reflected in the expected outcomes of therapy, the way stuttering is talked about, and the life experience of the person who stutters. However, childhood stuttering has less to do with the client's age than the degree to which he is troubled by his speech disfluencies. The typical child who stutters is marginally aware of the repetitions in his speech, happily communicating the events that occurred in his day despite the disfluencies in his speech production. The goal of therapy for this typical child is recovery from stuttering. We use caution not to react in an unfavorable or disapproving way to the child's speech and work to modify his speaking environments in ways known to facilitate fluency, rather than working directly on his stuttering.

But like adults, some children are painfully aware and frustrated by their inexplicable inability to speak like everyone else. Although recovery is still the expected outcome of therapy for these children, their strong reaction to their speech and sensitivity to the reactions of others in their environment necessitates a more direct approach to helping them better manage the physical aspects of their stuttering.

For adults, stuttering can become deeply intertwined in their identity. Recovery from stuttering is not the expected outcome and therapy, therefore, deals with learning to manage instances of stuttering, speaking in ways that promote natural fluency, and learning to cope more effectively with their feelings and perceptions of their stuttering. For adults, stuttering is a dramatic play that positions their speech against the reactions of society and their own expectations as a communicator. Their own instincts and natural reactions seemingly serve only to increase their stuttering, thereby eroding their confidence and self-esteem, while leaving them feeling helplessness.

The emotions of parents of children who stutter often run high as well. Parents often find themselves positioned between their role as their child's protector and not knowing how to help them. Watching your child suffer and worrying about his future can be very distressing. Educating parents and developing an active role for them to play in their child's therapy serves as a helpful and productive outlet for them and also strengthens the therapy team, producing a more satisfactory result.

Certain personal characteristics are helpful in those who treat stuttering, for it is not a straightforward, uncomplicated, or easy problem to resolve. Key ingredients include a penchant and excitement for mystery; a tolerance for ambiguity; the flexibility, maturity, self-confidence, and wisdom to know when to change course; hope and a vision for the future; and, certainly, patience. Stuttering is a disorder that engenders strong feelings and emotions. It is certainly intriguing. There are things about it that are very puzzling and cause us to appreciate the nuances and complexities of the process of speaking. There is excitement in the scientific and technologic advances, which bring us ever closer to discovering the roots of this communication problem. There is frustration in stuttering, on both sides of the therapy table. From the aggravation in the inability to verbally express yourself to the variable nature and severity of stuttering, clients and clinicians alike share strong feelings of frustration, disappointment, and sometimes defeat. But from the synergy that develops in joining together to overcome stuttering comes the strength for each to surmount these obstacles by working together.

Over many years I have come to appreciate stuttering for its complexity. Were it an easy problem to resolve, were to follow the same rules for everyone it afflicts, or were it predictable, I would likely have lost interest in it a long time ago. Helping others find a pathway to overcome their stuttering has provided many years of personal and professional satisfaction. As for stuttering, few other problems afford the opportunity to make such tangible differences in the lives of others. It is my hope that you will also discover and experience this in your work.

Gary J. Rentschler, PhD

Acknowledgments and Dedication

Stuttering has been a central feature in my life, shaping who I was growing up as a child, and then giving new direction to my life again after therapy as an adult. My stuttering went from being *despised* to being *accepted*—but never being *loved* (except for the wonderful people it has enabled me to meet). Growing up a child who stuttered was profoundly different from the experiences of most other children. Stuttering was an oppressor, a container that confined and defined who I was in the eyes of others and in my own mind. Therapy was a new beginning, a rebirth; the chance to emerge from the role in which I was cast to become who I really was. But the story is not the romanticized fairytale of a caterpillar transforming into a beautiful butterfly, but rather a journey of discoveries and realizations in a search of true self.

There is a lengthy list of people who have helped me along the way. Perhaps foremost are my speech therapist, Dr. Lewis K. Shupe, and my student clinician, Diane Krieger at the SUNY Buffalo Speech & Hearing Clinic; they taught me about my stuttering and gave me the tools to effectively manage it—a personal battle I now happily place in the "Personal Victories" column. Certainly, my family continues to be a core foundation of support in that they never made my stuttering an issue and treated me just like everyone else.

There are the many colleagues and friends who helped shape my opinions and thinking about stuttering over the years, who encouraged me to try new things, and who offered opportunities for me to grow professionally and personally.

There are, too, the many people whose lives have intersected with mine because of our stuttering. More than anyone, they have taught me about stuttering by sharing their insights and their struggles. They continue to open new perspectives and horizons in my appreciation for this disorder.

It's not easy being in a position of needing help; it's usually far more comfortable being the helper. Nonetheless, rewards come to both the helper and the person needing help, working together to find a means of resolving stuttering. Through this book I hope in some way to enable more people to become helpers and that more people who stutter will find a successful resolution to their problems from their help.

CHAPTER

1

Basic Clinical Skills for Stuttering Therapy

Learning about any area of speech pathology (or any discipline) is facilitated by understanding and sharing an orientation to the subject. The intent of this chapter is to establish a perspective for the reader and present a general guide to the process of stuttering therapy.

Among the important things to understand is that the orientation of stuttering therapy for children and therapy for adults are very different. Children in the early phases of stuttering have an opportunity for recovery and consequently the primary objective of therapy becomes facilitating that recovery. For older children, adolescents, and adults, stuttering is usually chronic and therapy seeks to provide a means of effectively managing their stuttering and learning to speak in a manner that promotes their natural speech fluency.

There are some fundamental clinical skills for clinicians working with people who stutter that are discussed in this chapter. To be able to better satisfy our "customers," it is important to understand their perspectives as they seek therapy and throughout the therapeutic process.

Chapter Outline

Introduction

People who stutter report that the single most important ingredient of their success in therapy is their clinician regardless of the treatment approach used. Although there are basic traits that characterize good clinicians, stuttering therapy demands some additional skill sets, broader insights, and a tolerance for ambiguity, uncertainty, and variability. These demands arise from the personal nature of the impact that stuttering represents and the variety of ways people who stutter react to it. For parents of children who stutter it stems from the fear of how stuttering might affect their child's future psychological well-being and social acceptance. For adolescents and adults who stutter, the impact is rooted in the degree to which stuttering can affect one as a person. Therefore, clinicians in stuttering therapy not only need to have good therapy skills, but also need to have strong counseling skills as well. Clinicians new to stuttering therapy usually underestimate the importance of counseling as an integral part of the treatment. Working with parents, the counseling consists of providing accurate, current information about stuttering, helping them problem-solve difficult situations, and facilitating their role in reaching therapy goals and advocating for their child. For adults who stutter, counseling includes changing feelings and attitudes, developing an accurate knowledge base, better managing their anxieties, and overcoming past (and current) difficult experiences with stuttering. Although experienced clinicians are prepared to deal with the speech aspects of stuttering, they often find the variability of stuttering and difficulties people who stutter have in managing their speech fluency to be frustrating and sometimes discouraging. The chapters that follow provide a rationale to help clinicians develop a philosophy of stuttering to guide their thinking, decision-making, and therapy planning. Clinicians new to stuttering therapy must understand the significance and impact of these psychological variables that contribute to the persistence of stuttering. These factors underscore the need for counseling as part of stuttering therapy, as these psychological reactions to stuttering (the anxiety, fears, beliefs, and emotions) are the bases of many of the associated difficulties.

A good way to appreciate the culture of stuttering is to become involved with a support group, such as Friends or the National Stuttering Association. Listening to the struggles faced by adults who stutter and the concerns of parents of children who stutter builds an appreciation for the impact of this disorder's impact in a way that is more personal and dramatic than just reading about it.

The treatment approaches for children who stutter and adults who stutter vary in significant ways. In the early stages of stuttering, it is important that caution be taken so that the child's awareness of the problem (particularly an awareness that something is different and wrong about how they speak) is minimized. Prior to becoming aware of stuttering, the child does not react to it. At this level of stuttering development, disfluencies are usually easy and effortless and the child shows little concern for his speech. But as his awareness grows, he attempts to speak in different ways to escape from his stuttering or avoid instances of stuttering. Speaking more quickly, beginning utterances abruptly, or using more muscular effort in articulating sounds are common ways people who stutter react to their disfluencies.

As awareness of the speech differences grows, the reactions to stuttering increase and the fear of stuttering emerges and becomes habitual. Later, the individual begins to think of himself as a communicator in different ways. Because instances of stuttering seem to be involuntary and uncontrollable, feelings of loss of power and helplessness commonly emerge. As others react to the unabated stuttering, feelings of embarrassment and sometimes shame develop. These feelings and experiences fuel fear and anxiety, which create greater muscle tension, and result in more stuttering. The cycle of stuttering spins and deepens. Speaking rituals develop; stuttering becomes a larger factor in making life decisions (large and small). Fully developed, one's self-concept and self-image as a communicator are affected, and the person thinks of himself as a person who stutters, someone unable to communicate easily or effectively. With adults, adolescents, and some children who stutter, approaches to therapy are directed at taking control of stuttering moments, learning speaking techniques that better parallel normal speech production, and learning to better cope with the feelings and emotions associated with their stuttering. Stuttering thus may be viewed from the perspective of the client's reaction to his speech. There are those (usually younger children) who demonstrate little awareness or concern (and hence minimal reaction to their stuttering) and those who are very concerned and purposefully react to it.

As a consequence, the therapeutic philosophy and approaches working with these separate perspectives of stuttering also differ. Chapters 2 and 3 present these two different approaches in greater detail. Each approach is based on certain beliefs about stuttering. Although a philosophy of treatment underlying stuttering therapy is offered in this book, clinicians are encouraged to develop their own philosophies, based on their beliefs, study, and experiences.

One of the frustrations in learning about this subject is that there are too few universal truths about stuttering. For each generalization made about stuttering, there is a person who stutters for whom the statement does not appear to hold true. There are people who stutter who do so when they sing; there are people who stutter for whom using a slow speaking rate or a metronome does not induce greater fluency. There are people who stutter less when talking to a large crowd than they do speaking to a single listener. Many generalizations about people who stutter and stuttering behaviors are put forward in this text. In the interest of ease of reading and writing this book, readers should be aware that exceptions to the generalizations are not acknowledged in every instance. Also, for the reader's and writer's ease, the author refers to people who stutter as "he" and clinicians as "she" in full recognition that there are women who stutter and men who are speech pathologists. The facts that more males than females stutter and that more women than men become speech pathologists are well known.

Getting Oriented

Stuttering therapy itself seems to be a rather polarizing topic: clinicians seem to either love it or hate it, with very few falling anywhere in between. The issues that make working with stuttering frustrating, aggravating, and challenging for clinicians are the very things that can make it interesting intellectually and a test of the clinician's skills. Developing an attitude of being open to change, embracing a challenge to one's skills, and embracing learning can become a tremendous advantage when working with this disorder. Expectations of a "right way" to treat stuttering, there being a perfect solution, or even anticipating the client making a steady progression of successes may not represent an optimal orientation for the stuttering therapy clinician. Stuttering therapy is as much an art as a science. It affects each individual and his family uniquely. There is much that remains unknown about stuttering and a great deal of folklore and misinformation; yet, the therapist is expected to be all-knowing, definitive, and upbeat about the prospects of therapy.

Learning about a client and how he is affected by stuttering is a continuing process of assimilating and accommodating new information. We begin with a hypothesis of the nature of the client's problem and modify it over time, either fitting new pieces of information into the existing structure of our knowledge or changing that structure to incorporate the new information that is discrepant with our understanding of the client. Meeting a person for the first time, we form an initial opinion from the characteristics we observe during our initial encounter. Over time, new information comes to light that can alter the way we perceive them and what we think of them. The longer the relationship and the more interactions we have with the client, the clearer the picture we develop and the stronger our opinions become. Consider our relationship with the client to be similar to that of making any new acquaintance. We form an initial impression in the first interaction but our knowledge, understanding, and opinions continue to evolve over time. At any point in time, we should be able to articulate our understanding of the client and his stuttering based on the assimilation and accommodation of new information over the period of time we know them. Over time, we learn to predict what the client might say or do given a specific circumstance, in the same way that you could predict what your mother would say if you were to start smoking or got a ticket for speeding. Predicting how the client will react gives us power in therapy. Clients' predictability comes from knowing them very well and understanding what they believe and how they think.

There are some speech pathologists who do not relish working with stuttering, some who "have to" work with it, but very few who are ambivalent about it. Many clinicians report that they are uncomfortable with stuttering because they are unsure of what to do and feel that they could make the problem worse instead of better. Stuttering constantly challenges what clinicians—even the experts—know and believe about the disorder. Stuttering is not commonly overcome quickly, so clinicians need extraordinary patience, persistence, and commitment. At the same time, they need to be a motivational force to push, and sometimes pull, clients through the process.

Many speech pathologists are surprised that much of stuttering therapy consists of counseling, educating the client and his parents, helping to resolve specific problems, and helping older clients to manage the psychosocial aspects of the disorder. For those who view stuttering therapy as working solely on aspects of the client's speech, this counseling component may not feel much like speech therapy. But at the advanced developmental stages of stuttering, much of the disorder is vested in the client's thoughts, fears, and beliefs about his stuttering. We see that these thoughts underlie the client's fears and anxieties, which increase muscular tension while speaking and precipitate stuttering.

Only working on the behavioral surface features of stuttering (the audible blocks, repetitions, and prolongations) is insufficient to manage the disfluencies at their source. In Chapter 3, the case is made that failing to address the client's thoughts, beliefs, and feelings does not result in a long-term resolution of his stuttering. Although on the surface it appears logical that the client's feelings about stuttering should disappear once he becomes a fluent speaker, experience has shown that this is not the case and, in fact, it likely increases the chance of relapse. Counseling includes building an adequate information base about stuttering so the client knows and better understands the nature of stuttering and the characteristics that define his experience with it. It also incorporates an understanding of how his thoughts and beliefs about stuttering impact the frequency of stuttering and the handicapping effects that result. Counseling also helps the client learn to better manage his fluency in stressful speaking situations. Thus, counseling plays a large role in therapy with adults and older children who are aware of their stuttering.

With younger children who are unaware and unconcerned about their stuttering, counseling with parents consists of educating, helping problem-solve, and supporting their role as parents of a stuttering child. As described in greater detail in Chapter 2, we can help parents by providing them with accurate information about stuttering and a model of stuttering that enables them to develop an understanding of their child's difficulties. This supports their role in the process of therapy by outlining areas in which they play a vital part. Clinicians find that this can facilitate more discussion about stuttering, and part of our goal in counseling is learning more about the child's and family's experience with it. In addition, parents often need to be prepared to look at their child's stuttering as a journey, rather than a short trip.

Counseling and providing therapy for people who stutter may require speech pathologists to "lead by following." The client (or client's parents) is a primary source of our information. Because each client's characteristics are unique and often differ greatly from others who stutter, clinicians need to become skilled at soliciting critical pieces of information about the client's stuttering over time, forming a mental picture of how this specific client fits the model of stuttering.

With the pressures and demands of a caseload and other work responsibilities, it often is easier to treat the patient without fully incorporating him into the process because it often seems to be more expedient for the clinician to direct the course of therapy. However, the client is more likely to become invested in his own therapy if he is made part of the process. It could be argued that this is an essential part of the therapy and, most assuredly, that it is the central part of the counseling. Either way, the client becomes more involved and more responsible for the treatment when he understands what will happen in therapy and is involved in making decisions. This subtly casts a greater weight of responsibility and investment in the process onto the client, whether they are adults or children, or their parents.

Communicating the overall treatment plan to the client could be considered a part of our counseling efforts. Keeping the client informed, and helping him understand his therapy, his current status in the overall plan, and what lies ahead in therapy, engage the client in his treatment. The clinician might think of this as an investment that will pay dividends later, as the therapy proceeds, and sow the seeds of longer term success.

Basic Clinical Skills

Therapy is about making changes: changes in motor movement, in brain functioning, and sometimes even in the way a patient thinks.

Stuttering therapy entails each of these components and the therapist's role is to facilitate changes in a client's communication as his guide, mentor, teacher, coach, or other means within the skill set of the clinician.

Certain techniques serve to enhance learning, for example, clearly stating the desired outcome of an activity and why it is important to the client. Obviating the goal and its importance allows the client to prepare himself for learning the specifics of that objective. Priming the client for what he is about to do enables him to make appropriate accommodations for the objective and heightens his attention to the kernel ingredients of the activity. Consider the difference between being told that a ball will be thrown to you and that you are expected to catch it, with just tossing a ball at someone unexpectedly and hoping he will catch it. In the first instance, in anticipation of what will happen, the individual can make whatever adjustments necessary to prepare for what he expects will happen; perhaps by putting down anything he might be holding in his hands and looking for the ball before it is thrown to him. The likelihood of success is enhanced greatly by first creating the expectation of what is to happen.

A related component is to explain the significance of the activity to the client's treatment. The clinician might say, *"In this next activity, we're going to practice using the easy onset technique on the first word of each sentence that you will read. I've noted that you often begin utterances rather abruptly in conversations; that leads to more stuttering. So I want you to begin by practicing in reading, where you can focus more on using the technique and less on formulating something to say, as one needs to do in a conversation."* Now the client understands not only what he will be asked to do, but also what it is intended to accomplish and why it is important to him.

Feedback

Providing feedback is a powerful teaching tool for the clinician. Feedback affords a crucial element for learning, from a perspective not otherwise available to the client. For example, all professional tennis players have a coach. In each case, the professional player could easily beat their coach in a game of tennis. So why have a coach? What can the coach offer to the player? The coach offers a perspective on the player's performance that the player cannot see from his own vantage point. The coach can see things that player cannot see himself, or that he is not aware of. In therapy, the clinician is the client's coach, able to offer feedback from a perspective to which the client is not attuned. With time, we need to train the client to be his own coach to the best of his abilities; but in therapy the clinician serves as the client's guide. The clinician might say, *"I noticed that at the beginning you caught yourself speeding up and then put the brakes on. But as the conversation went on your rate increased again. You need to stay vigilant longer, continuing to monitor your rate all the way through the conversation."* It appeared that the client was aware that he was speeding up initially, but the clinician observed that he hadn't stayed with it long enough. Had the client been aware of it at the time, he would likely have shown signs of trying to slow his rate.

The clinician's feedback is like the steering wheel in a car. It is used to direct the client's responses toward the desired destination or goal. Steering a car, the driver makes a continuous series of adjustments, some large and some small, in response to road conditions, or desired changes in direction, and to avoid obstacles along the way. The driver must always remain vigilant to successfully negotiate the obstacles in bringing the vehicle to the destination. In therapy, the client is the driver and the clinician the navigator; the clinician directs the driver around obstacles, through difficult conditions, and helps him avoid obstacles along the route to the final destination by giving him feedback along the way.

How much feedback does a client need? In the early stages of therapy or when teaching a new therapy technique, imagine that the client is driving blindfolded and relying on you to give him feedback. How often would you want feedback if you were driving blindfolded through the downtown area of a city? Would every 5 minutes be enough? Likely not. Every 30 seconds? At the very least! Would you only want to know when there was a pedestrian walking in front of the car or when you were approaching a stop light? Or would you want to know that everything was "good for the moment" as you proceeded? In the initial stages of therapy, clients need a lot of "steering," and not just when their responses are in some way inaccurate. They benefit from hearing that their productions were as you desire them to be as well. As a rule of thumb, give the client feedback, positive or corrective, every 30 seconds for the first 5 minutes of an activity. Continue at that rate if after that time he is still inaccurate. If he is successful, continue providing feedback once every minute or two. Keep the image of the blindfolded driver in mind to guide you in giving your client feedback.

The following is an example of giving guiding feedback:

Clinician: *"I'd like you to read each of the following sentences using a syllable stretch on the first sound of the first word of each sentence. Let's begin with the first sentence."*

Client: *"Brea-a-a-a-a-a-d is the foundation of every sandwich."*

Clinician: *"Great! You stretched the syllable just long enough."*

Client: *"The-e-e-e-e filling is important too."*

Client: *"Co-o-o-o-ndiments put zest in every bite."*

Clinician: *"That's it."*

Client: *"The-e-re are several types of bread to choose from."*

Clinician: *"I think that your stretch was too short; let's give that another try."*

Client: *"The-e-e-e-e-e-re are several types of bread to choose from."*

Clinician: *"Yes!"*

The clinician comments on both successful and unsuccessful responses. She instructs the client how to improve the poorer ones by identifying the features of the response to be changed and improved.

Data Collection

The clinician is responsible for collecting data to measure the client's performance level during therapeutic activities. The data help the clinician document the client's progress throughout the course of treatment and make necessary adjustments to specific activities so that they challenge, but do not overwhelm, the client's emerging fluency skills. Although the goal of therapy is improved fluency, the objective of therapy is for the client to use a new speaking techniques or "targets" in order to change his speaking behaviors and establish new speech patterns. What we are teaching is target use; speech fluency is the desired byproduct of using targets. As a consequence, we collect data on the frequency and accuracy of the client's target use, not the fluency that results. There is a good deal of variability in a client's fluency and clients commonly report having "good" and "bad" fluency days. Their variations, however, are not related to their target use; instead, they are part of the natural, day-to-day cycle of stuttering. As a consequence, collecting data on a client's fluency (instead of his target use) would reflect these natural variations rather than the client's ability to use his targets. This would not be an accurate measurement of his success in therapy, but rather his "luck" in being fluent. Our therapy is "luck," it is hard work and we need to measure what is within the client's control; his ability to use targets. The clinician's data must reflect the client's accuracy in using targets, rather than how fluent he was. We look for fluency to be a byproduct of target use, but it is also a reflection of "the forces of fate" that are beyond our control. Therefore, measuring the client's fluency is an unreliable measurement of the client's performance in therapy. Count the client's *target use*, not his fluency.

Types of Responses in Counseling

Counseling is an integral part of the therapeutic process in resolving stuttering; therapy is not just practicing speech techniques. The most effective counseling is usually client centered. The clinician or counselor probes to learn the issues that arise from the client before responding. Like speech therapy, counseling has a skill set of its own. Although counseling is a part of most patient interactions, regardless of the disorder, it plays a very fundamental role in stuttering therapy. Training in counseling is included in the curriculum at some university speech-language pathology programs. Stuttering therapy can require a clinician to be well versed in counseling techniques. In counseling, Luterman (2008) presents ways of encouraging clients to interact. The following are brief examples of types of responses a clinician may use when counseling a client during sessions:

- **Content Response:** Information is communicated that is factual, straightforward, and brief. Typically, an answer to a direct question or when providing factual information for the client is the desired goal.
  Example: *"Many who stutter may have a family history of stuttering. There is now evidence that genetics plays a role."*
- **Counter Question:** People often don't want advice, but seek confirmation of their position or decision. Clients often don't learn from advice and it doesn't promote self-reliance in making decisions. Questioning a client's expressed beliefs

is a means of helping them question themselves. Counterquestioning moves the relationship beyond an initial or information exchange stage. A counterquestion implies that the client may need to consider another perspective without stating that his position is wrong.
Example: *"If that was true, do you think others in your office feel that way too?"*

- **Affect Response:** This form of reply helps the clinician see the world as the client does and reflect his feelings back to him. Accurate reflections make the client feel that he is understood. Inaccurate reflections force the client to clarify his position and thereby the clinician's understanding.
Example: *"That must have been an embarrassment for you at the party."*
- **Reframing:** Reframing is finding an alternative explanation that makes an event seem somehow more acceptable, offering a perspective that is both believable and enables the client to discover a new, more palatable explanation of an event. Good reframing resonates with the client and gives him a jolt of satisfaction.
Example: *"Perhaps he commented about your stuttering because he was surprised and didn't expect your speech to be different?"*
- **Sharing Self:** Sharing your personal insights and experiences enables clients to view the clinician as human and imperfect, just as they view themselves. This usually results in deepening and enhancing the therapeutic relationship. The information is shared in a way that enables a client to view his flaws with the same dignity as the clinician.
Example: *"When I was introducing my wife to a friend I got stuck because I couldn't remember her name at the minute and, boy, she never let me forget it!"*
- **Affirmations:** Sometimes clients need someone to be a positive sounding board for their ideas. The clinician may use the power and wisdom to say nothing new; only assuring the client that he has been heard.
Example: *"Indeed, that wasn't your best attempt; I can see why you are upset."*
- **Silence:** Saying nothing or not responding to the client's utterance is a technique that implies that the client should talk more and that the clinician wants and expects additional information will be forthcoming. There are a number of different types of silence responses:
  - **Embarrassed Silence:** In the initial stages of the relationship, a tolerance for silence establishes a degree of power for the clinician and serves to diminish familiarity.
  Example: Clinician: *"What do you think other people think when you stutter?"* Client: *"I don't know."* The clinician stares at the client in silence waiting for him to say more.
  - **Changing the Topic:** Often, troducing a different topic. The clinician needs to guide the interaction back to the main topic by ignoring the client's comments or acknowledging the new topic, promising to return to it at an appropriate time.
  Example: Client: *". . . and my co-workers never get chastised for taking long*

breaks; only me!" Clinician: *"Whoa! We were talking about how hard it is to speak fluently with your boss; let's tackle the issue of taking long breaks another time."*

- **Reflective Silence:** When a topic is particularly emotionally laden, silence may be used to allow the client time to think and reflect on what has been said. The client may be asked to share his reflections after several moments.
- **Termination Silence:** As approaches the end of the session approaches, the clinician may become quieter and less interactive as a means of signaling the conclusion.

Skillful use of these responses takes time and practice to master. Keep in mind, the goal is to find productive ways to facilitate clients' willingness to contribute to their own care. Counseling is part of the art of therapy. It allows the clinician to learn how to motivate the client, persuade him to entertain new perspectives, and overcome the obstacles that inevitably arise as part of therapy. Counseling is more of an art than a science, but it is the backbone supporting the treatment process. Understanding the client's views on his stuttering enables the clinician to encourage his efforts more effectively. Knowing how he feels and how these feelings came about can help the clinician avoid making painful mistakes in therapy. Knowing and understanding the client is a fundamental element to successful therapy.

Treatment Basics

Like therapy for any communicative disorder, therapeutic activities in stuttering therapy play a central role in clinical teaching and learning. Activities provide a clinical environment intended to enable the client to practice a specific skill while various elements and parameters are manipulated to adjust to the difficulty of the task. Task difficulty is determined by the success rate attained by the client engaged in the activity. There usually are several dimensions to each activity that serve as tools for the clinician to modify it in order to appropriately challenge the client. The challenge must be sufficient to allow the client a reasonable level of success. In other words, an activity should be neither too difficult nor too easy to optimally facilitate the client's learning. A success rate of 75% to 90% generally is considered to be optimal. If the client's level of performance is lower, consider changing one parameter to make the activity less difficult. If the client is getting more than 90% correct, it usually is prudent to make the activity harder or to move on to another, more difficult activity.

The clinician has the responsibility to move her client through therapy as quickly as possible. Spending too much time in therapy on tasks in which the client is already successful may not be using time most effectively. However, most clients benefit from activities designed to keep existing skills sharp; this promotes carryover and confidence. Therefore, a good compromise may be to assign mastered activities as homework or use them as a warm-up at the beginning of the session.

Parameters

The level of challenge of most stuttering therapy activities can be manipulated by a variety of factors, which include the physical speaking environment, the complexity of the utterances, and the degree of difficulty of the task as perceived by the client.

The Speaking Environment

The effect of the speaking environment varies widely among people who stutter. Generally, clients who stutter experience more difficulty talking on the phone, giving presentations, speaking to authority figures, and introducing themselves to strangers. On the other end of the continuum, most who stutter report that their stuttering is greatly diminished when they speak when alone or when speaking in unison with someone else, while reading aloud, or when whispering or singing. Again, individual circumstances vary, so it is important to work with the client to determine the critical variables characteristic of his specific speaking environments.

Additionally, many who stutter find specific words (their name, for example), sounds, or particular communication partners to be examples of when the frequency of their stuttering increases. These fears are often learned. You likely will observe many examples of the client being able to say his name fluently or articulate specific sounds he has identified as being difficult. This is indicative of the complexity and variability of stuttering and should not be used as an example to contradict the client's beliefs. Analogously, it is a commonly held belief that it snows (in the northern United States) in the winter. It doesn't snow every day, but the belief still stands that the winter season is characterized by snowfall. Just because it does not snow every day does not mean that winter is not snow season. Sometimes fluency just happens; therapy helps the client to create his own fluency instead. Consequently, therapy teaches the client to use speech targets for this purpose. But therapy also needs to respect the client's beliefs, whether they are accurate or inaccurate. The client's perception is his reality; not to respect the client's beliefs usually serves to distance the clinician from the client. But therapy can be an effective tool to alter the client's beliefs.

> **Clinical Example:** From past experiences, many clients believe that people will ridicule or make fun of them when they find out about their stuttering. As a consequence, the clinician's suggestion that clients tell new acquaintances that they stutter usually is not well received. To their surprise, clients willing to try the suggestion most often are met not with ridicule but with a sincere, intellectual curiosity of stuttering. Other clients have been surprised to find their new acquaintance to be interested in knowing what they might do to help! Appreciating the subtle difference between telling someone about his stuttering and stuttering without acknowledging it, enables the client to change his belief about needing to keep it hidden.

Clients often demonstrate subtle nuances in the degree of difficulty in specific situations, which helps the clinician adjust the level of difficulty of some activities to the appropriate degree of challenge. The telephone is a good example. Telephone calls can be made in various ways: just holding the receiver to the ear (without actually dialing); speaking phone-to-phone with the clinician while both are in the same room; calling a familiar person in the clinic; calling a store and asking their hours of operation; making a dinner reservation (leaving your name and callback number); canceling the reservation later; calling Victoria's Secret asking for gift suggestions for a spouse or friend; calling for information about an item on Craigslist; calling someone familiar and reading them information over the telephone, and so on. There are individual differences among clients in the degree of difficulty that they perceive these specific activities as being. Work with the client and discuss his perceptions of these various iterations of telephone calling to construct a hierarchy of difficult situations. Start on the "easy" end of the continuum and work up to the most difficult situation. Expect inconsistency in client performance levels, but do not let that deter the overall direction of your work.

Much of what makes a speaking situation difficult for the client comes from thoughts and beliefs that have developed over time. A surprising number of beliefs may have stemmed from childhood and lingered on or even grown over the course of time. For some who stutter, each incidence of stuttering is accompanied by a flashback to that first embarrassing moment of stuttering and a synthesis of other events that grew from it. Some believe that the original incident may remain an open wound because the client was not able to soothe his feelings in childhood with the coping skills he had at the time. The painful experience is covered over and has not been revisited because the pain is too great. Left unattended the incident may fester. Re-examining the original episode as an adult, with adult coping skills, can go a long way to promote healing and overcome the difficult feelings, finally bringing to it a degree of closure.

Utterance Complexity

There are at least three parameters of complexity that can influence the fluency of an utterance. They include the coordination of speech motor movements required, the onset of an utterance, and the intricacy of the speaking process involved.

Some who stutter appear to have less accurate or less precise motor speech and articulation skills, even as adults. Sometimes a few sounds (particularly sounds that require more articulatory accuracy or are more complex to produce, like /s/, /th/, or /r/) can be slightly "slurred" or imprecise. Other signs include speaking inappropriately loudly for a specific communicative context. Usually, slowing the rate of speech results in at least a slight improvement in speech accuracy and fluency. The slower rate might be a more optimal speed for the client's motor system to execute speech. The slower rate also enables the speaker more time to put thoughts into words, find the words that accurately reflect his thoughts, program motor movements for speaking, and enable more time to improve the accuracy of movements, and more time to monitor the result.

Much of the complexity of speaking is seen at the very initiation of speech, at the precise moment when the client transitions from silence to speaking. We see that a very high percentage of disfluencies occur at the onset of speech, so this is a place to focus use of the appropriate speech target. At this precise moment, the speaker changes his breathing from inhalation to exhalation and voice onset follows very shortly thereafter, followed by movements of the oral structures to form the sounds. The timing is very precise and even though, for most speakers, this is a highly practiced (and successful) motor routine, for the person who stutters, it is complicated by the fear that he will be unsuccessful and stuttering will result. Some categories of sounds, such as plosives, can be more problematic as they are begun by occluding the breath stream in order to build intraoral breath pressure—this sometimes feels akin to stuttering itself. As anxiety and worry increase, so does muscle tension, heightening the risk of an awkward start to the utterance.

When speaking is made less complex, there is greater fluency. For example, removing just the element of voicing (as in whispering) frequently increases fluency. Thus, when the client whispers, he stutters less. When the client does not need to generate the content of his speech (for instance, when he reads a script aloud or parrots what someone else says), stuttering often decreases. Similarly, even reducing loudness usually can benefit fluency. Also, when the rhythm and melody of speech is prescribed (like in a song) or speaking to the beat of a drum, stuttering can decrease dramatically.

Manipulating the variables discussed above helps to manage the degree of challenge of activities. However, of all the possible permutations of these variables, some may not be perceived as being socially appropriate by the client, for example, singing his name when introducing himself. Suggesting he do so would likely elicit more resistance from the client. However, intentionally speaking more softly is much less likely to be considered inappropriate. Be sure to work with the client to actively recruit and encourage his participation. But remember that medicine that doesn't taste good is not necessarily bad for you. Part of the clinician's job is to weigh the potential benefits against the client's resistances to the prescribed activities; this is not always an easy determination to make.

Client Perceptions

It is useful to begin therapy by discussing aspects of stuttering that the client has found to be more difficult and challenging. Typically, clients report some specific sounds, words, and speaking situations as being more difficult than others. It is very common for people who stutter to report that their own name is among the most difficult of words to say fluently.

A client's perception of difficulty is influenced strongly by his learning throughout the time that he has stuttered. A single embarrassing incident of stuttering on a particular sound or word can begin the thought that that word will be more difficult to say than others. It is eliciting the emotion (embarrassment in this instance) that makes the memory more powerful, effectively punctuating the recollection of the incident. The client's beliefs are very strong and he often feels the need to do something extra to avoid having a disfluency again. As a result, people who stutter typically speed up their speaking rate or use more force when articulating the feared sound or word, as a means of overcoming it. Ironically, this reaction usually increases, rather than decreases, the likelihood of being disfluent. Other compensatory behaviors include abruptly initiating the feared word or taking a noticeable, sudden inhalation of air just prior to uttering the feared word.

Working with the client to establish a hierarchy of perceived difficulty of speaking situations and environments helps the clinician to structure therapy activities and adjust their level of difficulty. Subtleties in designing and structuring activities can have a profound influence on the client's success.

Response Rate

Another means of measuring the effectiveness of an activity is the response rate it generates. How many responses does the activity yield from the client per minute? Among other things, speaking is a motor skill and like any motor skill, it can improve with practice. Generally, more practice results in more improvement and better performance. This is not necessarily true, however, when we look at rate of speaking. In general, the slower, the more successful. In terms of improving most aspects of speech targets; the more practice the better. It is intuitive that an activity that yields more practice opportunities should produce better results faster, and thus be more desirable. Therefore, an activity that generates 15 responses per minute is superior to one that yields only 3 per minute. But, although there are other means of gauging an activity, the number of responses generated is an easy target for the clinician to shoot for.

Utility

Clients generally participate more fully when they can see the relevance of the activity in their daily life. Thus, playing word games like "Taboo" can be perceived as being "less therapeutic" and less valuable than having the client practice introducing himself to others or just making conversation with someone new. Clients generally are aware of their need to improve social communication skills and tend to value activities such as these more than playing games.

Other useful activities include making phone calls, giving brief (2- to 3-minute) presentations or monologues, instructing or explaining how to do something (like hooking up a wireless printer or something else in the client's skill set), giving directions to a specific destination, discussing pictures from a trip or vacation, or describing the advantages or disadvantages of a particular car or smartphone. Consider things that the client likely might be called on to do in his environment at work, school, and at home. These are situations that comprise the client's life and he will see the relevance in practicing and rehearsing them.

> **Clinical Insight:** Be wise to your client. Clients frequently will profess to prefer one activity over another because, in actuality, one activity may be easier in the sense of being less confrontational or less threatening to him. Some clients will tell you that they do not need to practice telephone calls because making calls is not problematic for them, when in reality they may be trying to avoid making calls because it is so difficult.

First Session Advice

Stuttering is an exceedingly difficult and often frustrating problem to treat because progress often seems slow. Clients resist changing behaviors, and the frequency of stuttering itself is so variable. Many clinicians are somewhat apprehensive about working with clients who stutter; they often fear they will make the stuttering worse and are unsure of what to do. A few suggestions are offered to assist in your first therapeutic encounters.

Focus on Speech Therapy First

The point has been made that stuttering therapy deals with both speech behaviors and the psychodynamic aspects that result from them. Start with the speech behaviors. Having a reliable speech technique to help manage stuttering is an invaluable tool for clients and is the backbone of effective therapy with adolescents and adults. New clients are unlikely to share much of their feelings and emotions about stuttering with any clinician; it often takes time to get to know someone and trust them enough to open up about the personal details of their problem. As clients become better able to manage their stuttering and see progress in therapy, they become more open to talking about how stuttering has impacted their lives and share their feelings and beliefs about their stuttering.

Have a Solid Rationale for What You Do

Know what you are doing, and why, in each component of your therapy session. The best therapy is usually "client-centered"; if you thoroughly understand your objective, making the adjustments and alterations based on your client's individual needs will be much easier. One way of doing this is to develop a philosophy of the disorder of stuttering that you are treating. The information in this book is presented based on a philosophy; however, clinicians are encouraged to develop their own philosophy based on their beliefs, experiences, and findings from research studies. Clinicians earn credibility and the client's respect by being able to explain the rationale for what they ask the client to do. An educated client will progress more rapidly and sustain the gains he makes longer if he understands what he is doing and why.

Keep Perspective

Remember above all that you are working with a *person* who stutters, not just a speech problem. Stuttering can have a significant impact on a person's life and his family and friends. That's the important part. Stuttering is a personal problem that impacts the way the individual sees himself and how others view him as well. That is what makes stuttering therapy so satisfying; the result is not just better speech fluency, it is helping someone realize their dreams in every facet of their life and all that they do. How many jobs afford that kind of personal satisfaction?

First Session Accomplishments

The points below are offered to help guide clinicians toward goals for themselves in early therapy sessions. By the conclusion of the first session you should:

- **Be able to describe the client's stuttering behaviors.** Know what you are working with. List the types of disfluencies the client displays, words and sounds that give him difficulty, and observe secondary characteristics, and other aberrant characteristics of the client's speech. Share your observations with the client (or parents of the child who stutters). This is a means of establishing an open, objective attitude when dealing with stuttering in therapy and helps begin to educate the client about aspects of the client's stuttering of which he might not yet be aware. Talking about stuttering openly communicates not only that you are knowledgeable and experienced, but that stuttering is something that can be discussed in a nonpejorative way; this is how a therapeutic relationship works successfully. To know and better understand the stuttering, the clinician should be able to imitate the client's stuttering (but not necessarily in front of the client). If you can imitate the way the client stutters it demonstrates that you understand what is happening.
- **Establish a "down-to-business" tone for your session right from the start rather than starting with a casual, social conversation.** Clients pay for therapy, usually by the hour. Show them that every minute of therapy time matters. Imagine a plumber coming to your house, charging by the hour, and chit-chatting about his children! Should you be paying the plumber to provide you with updates about his family or fix your drain? Respect the client's time and maximize the effectiveness of your therapy by staying focused on the client's stuttering. Unlike personal relationships that are based on sharing information about family and other aspects of life, a therapeutic relationship needs to be focused squarely on the client's problem. The client will both like and respect you for valuing your time together. For example, the clinician might say, *"Hey Tom, nice to see you this week. Let's go right back to the room and get started. I'm anxious to hear how your speech targets worked in your presentation last Friday."*
- **Learn what your client needs and wants to accomplish in therapy.** Clinicians entering a therapeutic relationship with preconceived ideas of what a patient wants from therapy may not be doing their best for the client. If you ask, most clients will tell you what they want from therapy. Sometimes therapy is not able to give them what they want and it's important to let that be known from the onset. By analogy, going to the hair salon expecting that a haircut will make you look like a specific movie star (e.g., Keira Knightly) will likely end in disappointment. If the hairdresser discussed that with you before your cut, you are allowed time to alter your expectations to something more realistic. When a client expects effortless fluency to result from their therapy, it could be argued that proceeding under that impression might not be fair to the client and almost will certainly lead to disappointment with your work. Clinician's may wish

to speak openly and honestly to clients about feasible functional outcomes of therapy, such as being able to confidently give a presentation or being able to make a phone call while managing fluency. These outcomes are possible and are a more realistic way to begin shaping the client's expectations from therapy, and his overall satisfaction with the experience. Along the way, clients will learn to be more accepting of some stuttering in their speech. The client will also learn fluency-compatible speaking techniques and ways of better managing his speaking anxieties. Setting realistic expectations enhances client satisfaction and his appreciation of your efforts.

- **Be clear that *the client* is responsible for making the changes to his speech.** The clinician's role is as a guide or mentor. In educational terms, you cannot make someone learn, you can only teach them what to do. Learning requires action by the client. Therefore, the clinician's role is to teach the client by leading him to make specific changes by providing him with information, instruction, and opportunities through guided practice. We communicate the client's responsibility by using language that denotes the client's need for action in order to make changes. We reinforce this idea in our orientation toward problem-solving and planning and implementing his therapy. The clinician can only show the client what to do; the client's responsibility is in doing it.
- **Provide daily assignments that require some form of verification.** Stuttering cannot be resolved just by working in the therapy room. It is essential that the client carry his therapy techniques into all other aspects of his world. Too often clients report that they are fluent only in the therapy room. This leads them to think that our therapy does not work or is ineffective for them. For some clients, the leap from practicing speaking techniques in therapy to using them in the office or with friends is too great, and as a result they do not attempt it at all. Working with the client to determine what he feels he is realistically able and willing to do in other environments is a critical component in getting the client to complete homework. There sometimes is a fine balance between pushing the client too hard and increasing the likelihood that he will complete assignments. Working with the client to problem-solve may be a way of resolving this issue. Having the client suggest times or situations in which he feels he would be able to complete assignments serves both the goals of the client and the clinician. It also reinforces the idea that the client is responsible for making change. Including him in the decision-making process builds both a feeling of trust and responsibility.

  A means of verifying completion can also enhance the likelihood of completing assignments. For example, at meetings of weight loss groups, a "weigh-in" is a tremendously motivating factor. Knowing that "the scale doesn't lie" and that your efforts will be reported to others is very "inspirational." Construct a means for the client to report on homework assignments; perhaps by E-mail, logs, journaling, leaving phone messages, or discussing it at the next session. This provides more motivation for clients to actually do what is expected of them.

Things to Avoid

In your first and subsequent therapy sessions, try to:

- **Avoid focusing on counting disfluencies.** Therapy is about using speech targets. Fluency is a byproduct of using those targets. Fluency is sometimes spontaneous or "lucky." We cannot teach clients to be lucky; we can only teach them to use targets. Counting disfluencies misses the point of our instruction. In the same way, commenting on the client's fluency sends the wrong message. We instruct clients to use speech targets (techniques) as the primarily focus of their therapy. Therefore, it is the client's target use that we should count and need to provide feedback on.
- **Avoid wasting precious treatment time.** Therapy time is valuable and expensive and the client's time needs to be respected. Most people spend more time watching television commercials each week than they spend with you in therapy. You need to make an impact in each session. We are ethically obligated to move clients through therapy as quickly as they are able to progress. Clients feel respected when their time and expenditures are valued. In the process, the perception of the clinician as being 'very effective' is also enhanced.
- **Avoid focusing on yourself.** New clinicians usually want their clients to like them. It's our job to help the client, and that's where the focus needs to be aimed. In doing your job, the client will like you, but our paramount objective is to help the patient. You may have had a teacher in high school that you did not like so much at the time. But looking back afterward, you might acknowledge that he or she was a good teacher because she helped you learn by giving you what you needed. And sometimes what you needed might have been "a kick in the seat of the pants!" Your client doesn't have to like you for you to be a good speech pathologist. They aren't paying to have a friend; they are paying to be helped. In nearly all cases, if you can help them, they will like you.
- **For new clinicians, focusing on the client instead of yourself will help you be less nervous.** Worrying about what you will do, what the client will think of you, or what to do if something goes wrong just heightens your anxiety. A little anxiety is good; it indicates that you want to do a good job; if you didn't care, you wouldn't be anxious. Concentrating on the client and thinking about his needs and how to make him feel comfortable, shifts the focus from your anxiety to something more productive.

Meeting the Client for the First Time

The initial meeting with any client usually seems to be the most difficult because the "unknowns" are much greater than the "knowns." First impressions are important, but it takes time for a therapeutic relationship to develop. Be organized, set your agenda, be direct and speak authoritatively, and enjoy this new clinical challenge. People form a first impression of you in 7 seconds. Consider the impression that you want to make and think about how best to use your 7 seconds!

Here are some thoughts about managing the first interaction with a client.

- Set a businesslike tone by seeing the client as soon as they are ready, after they've taken care of any paperwork, signed forms, and any other procedures followed at your clinic. Be punctual.
- Introduce yourself and briefly explain your plans for today's visit. Then escort them to the treatment room, be seated, and get started.
- Generally speaking, beginning by asking an open-ended question about what brings the client to the clinic will reveal the *client's reason* for the meeting and what he hopes to accomplish from the visit. Be sure that the first meeting concludes by responding directly to the client's initial statement of the purpose of the appointment. This helps to ensure that the client will feel satisfied in achieving his initial goal. Even if the actual result of the meeting leads in a direction different than was initially sought by the client, the clinician should recap and explain how and why the "detour" was necessary.
- Share your thinking with the client throughout the meeting. Educate him by providing factual information and sharing your clinical experiences as the conversation continues. This affords the client the opportunity to acknowledge or rebut your suggestions, which will likely save time in the long run. It also is an integral part of educating the client.
- Be direct without being offensive. Talk about stuttering openly and objectively, just like you want the client to do. "Tip-toeing" around the topic only makes it seem somehow worse or more ominous than it actually is. Show the client how you think about stuttering by the words you choose and the manner in which you speak about it.
- Give the client enough opportunity to talk, letting you know his feelings, perceptions, and the information he has acquired about stuttering. This can be critical in understanding his current status and motivating him later in therapy.
- End the session by providing a review the accomplishments of the first meeting, a list of things still needing to be accomplished in future sessions, a brief statement about what is intended for next week, and what the client could do to begin working on his stuttering until the next meeting.

Another Perspective of Therapy

A different way to think about stuttering therapy is to consider the three elements that comprise the overall process: Information Gathering, Fluency Building, and Structuring for Continuing Success. This perspective is based on the following assumptions:

- **People who stutter usually lack objectivity in evaluating their stuttering; they are emotionally involved.** Most have acquired misinformation or have distorted perceptions about their stuttering. Therefore, establishing a good stuttering information base is an important fundamental step.

- **There are many approaches to building fluent speech; no single approach appears to work best for everyone.** Try not to get bogged down in a specific theory or a specific way to treat stuttering; be flexible and open to trying different things. The techniques used are probably less important than the clinician's ability to encourage and motivate the client to change his speaking habits in the directions that enhance his fluency.
- **Rebuilding attitudes and repairing feelings are important components of constructing a foundation for long-term success and continuing improvement.** Many have gained fluency only to lose it later. Others struggle to be able to change their habitual speaking patterns and find implementing therapy techniques to be a challenging endeavor.

Information Gathering

It is important to learn general information and specific facts about the normal processes of speaking, and how stuttering differs. There is considerable misinformation about the nature and causes of stuttering, which often serves to needlessly confuse and complicate the client's understanding of his difficulties and cope more successfully with stuttering. Knowledge is power, particularly in stuttering therapy.

Clients need to be able to identify the specifics of their own stuttering as well as recognize how their disfluencies differ from the normal speaking processes. An early and continuing focus of therapy needs to deal with developing this knowledge and building the client's vocabulary as it relates to speech production and stuttering. Later, clients can compare the way they stutter to others who stutter. Group therapy sessions or videos of others who stutter are instrumental in this endeavor. The initial goals of this process may be accomplished by clients learning to:

- Identify the core behaviors of their stuttering and how it differs from and interferes with fluent speech production.
- Recognize secondary stuttering characteristics as they relate to core behaviors of stuttering by being able to identify instances and describe the characteristics of these behavior patterns.
- Articulate their feelings, attitudes, and beliefs about stuttering and recognize the impact on muscle tension and movement control. Rebuilding attitudes and repairing feelings are important components of laying a foundation for long-term success and continuing improvement. Many have attained fluency only to lose it later. Others struggle to be able to change habitual speaking patterns and find implementing therapy techniques to be a real challenge. The clinician might initiate this topic by saying, *"It's common for clients to relapse at some point after therapy. In my experience this comes about when the rigorous practice required during therapy fades and when old feelings about stuttering creep back into the picture having not been completely resolved. We've talked about how those speaking anxieties increase*

muscle tension and enhance the likelihood of stuttering. This is why discussing your feelings about stuttering is so important. I know that that part of therapy has not always been easy, but I have found it to be a vital component in maintaining the fluency that you've worked so hard to attain. I hope we can continue exploring those feelings and working on ways to deal with them effectively."

Building Fluency

Clients need tools to help them change their habitual speaking patterns and develop new behaviors that enable them to manage their stuttering and speak in ways that optimize their fluency. In the past, their attempts to control stuttering have resulted in maladaptive habit patterns from which they are unable to deviate. Change is difficult because these maladaptive behaviors are produced in a mental state of fear and anxiety. The clinician provides different, more productive speaking techniques (targets) designed to be more compatible with the goal of fluent speech production. The fluency tools chosen need to be both effective in producing fluency and acceptable to the client. Even though they result in fluent speech, many clients object to using fluency targets outside the clinic room because they perceive that they will still sound different from other speakers; they therefore find the target unacceptable.

- In general, regardless of which fluency tool is utilized, the instructional paradigm for gaining control over stuttering and developing fluency patterning progresses through the stages of:

  Identifying → Modifying → Controlling and Shaping Fluency

  Clients must first identify (and be able to describe) disfluencies accurately and objectively. Next they learn to modify their habitual speech behaviors by substituting new speaking techniques for the old, disfluent ones. Gradually, they become adept at controlling their disfluencies and implementing new speaking behaviors with greater ease in order to manage their fluency.
- In another dimension, clients can become desensitized to the fear of speaking and the fear of stuttering. Eventually, this leads to readjusting their perceptions of themselves as a person who stutters and their success as a communicator. Concurrently, the speaking techniques become better integrated and more habituated.
- The client needs to understand and accept responsibility for speaking fluently and for making changes in how they speak.

Structuring for Continuing Success

There probably are as many reasons for fluency therapy to be unsuccessful as there are people who stutter. Relapse is very common, and therefore effective treatment programs must work to develop self-rescue skills and prepare clients for the relapses and setbacks that are likely to occur in the future. Adolescent and adult clients need to accept that their stuttering will always be with them as they are unlikely to recover at this point in their life. The following advice, therefore, might be useful for all clients who stutter:

- **Preparation**—Use focused, controlled speech as you enter difficult speaking situations; don't wait for "disaster" to happen, then try to recover. Be prepared; take the initiative by planning to be fluent by using speech targets, especially on the first utterances.
- **Attitude**—Think about speaking as being rewarding. Find satisfaction in communicating orally and define your success in terms of the information communicated, rather than the fluency of the spoken message. People do hear what you say, even when you stutter.
- **Challenges**—Actively seek out new speaking situations to continue to challenge your current speaking skills and develop new ones. Be willing to take risks. Like typing on a keyboard, the more often skills are practiced, the better they become. The less often they are used, the "rustier" and more dysfunctional they grow to be.
- **Confidence**—A sense of self-assurance while speaking is within the speaker's grasp. Cultivate a speaking personality and a sense of self. Add spontaneity by increasing inflection and intonation as more confidence is gained and more fluency develops. Learn to reflect your new persona as a successful communicator.
- **Relapse**—In life, as in stuttering, not every day is going to be a good day. Develop a plan in preparation for bad speaking days by networking with others who stutter. Become active in support groups. Be self-reliant by being your own speech coach and advocate. The measure of your success in not just how fluent you are, but what you do when you become disfluent.

Stuttering is a complex problem with many facets. Adolescents and adults who stutter come to learn many negative things about their stuttering, and most internalize these lessons. The process of becoming a successful communicator is lengthy and challenging.

Clients Who Have Had Therapy Before

Perhaps more than other communication disorders, clinical failures and relapse appear to be a common and unfortunate reality for those who stutter. Many adolescents and adults in therapy today have had therapy before, and for numerous reasons, they have returned. The disappointment, frustration, and feelings of failure and even anger, among many who stutter is easily understood.

There are few limits in finding sources of blame for relapse. But no matter the cause, it is the person who stutters who must assume responsibility for his recovery. Some clients come to therapy seeking to be "fixed," rather than understanding that they must actively effect their own fluency. Assuming responsibility for fluency is a fundamental tenet of successful therapy outcomes. However, the clinician's work is not complete until preparations for setbacks have been a part of the treatment program. Even at the end of therapy, many clients have not fully overcome the effects of their feelings and emotions about stuttering. If these feelings and emotions are not addressed in therapy, over time they will re-emerge and shake the client's confidence, often leading to an increase and the eventual return of their stuttering.

Many people who stutter have become soured to the prospect of therapy because of previous unsuccessful clinical encounters or clinicians who were less competent in treating the disorder. Some hold strong feelings of contempt for all speech-language pathologists as a result. Overcoming these feelings requires the clinician to demonstrate a degree of self-confidence and optimism while acknowledging the client's feelings. Experienced, successful fluency clinicians help the client to be cognizant of the obstacles yet to be overcome, the differences between his current performance and what is required, and the encouragement and motivation to make this treatment attempt successful.

Assessing the attitude of the client is important in understanding their perspective on treatment and learning about their previous attempts in therapy. Ham (1999) discussed some attitudes commonly held by people who stutter. These attitudes are paraphrased and elaborated upon below:

- **The Perfectionist:** For some who stutter, nothing is acceptable but being totally, 100% fluent. The content of an utterance is of far lesser importance. There is a very strong sensitivity and total rejection of any disfluency, and great discomfort in being in the presence of others who stutter. Perfectionism may be a predictable result of the criticism they have received for stuttering. To compensate, sadly, the feeling develops that they cannot allow even one disfluency to be considered a normal speaker.
- **Either/Or:** This patient sees in black or white, without acknowledging shades of grey between. Something is either "good" or "bad," and usually at an extreme. There is only success or failure with no sense of making progress by lessening or minimizing stuttering. A form of perfectionism, this client usually focuses on what he did wrong and is unable to credit himself for the parts of his performance that were good.
- **Yes, But:** Clients sometimes express superficial agreement with the clinician's perspective, but only make a token effort to implement their suggestions. *"I'll try it, but I couldn't do that outside the clinic." "I see that it might work for Tom, but it won't work for me."* This resistance often is based in fear, uncertainty, and insecurity. The client wants to feel like he is cooperating with his clinician, but at the same time his actions belie his words.
- **Prove It:** Rather than demonstrate his flexibility to think in new and different ways, this client offers resistance by requesting proof of ideas or concepts when it is impossible to offer them. These clients are usually rather dogmatic in their beliefs and like "Yes, but" clients, they are not truly invested in their clinician. Instead, they feel defeated and are convinced that they somehow are different from others who stutter, a special case. Some are afraid to try, feeling that therapy may be their last option. If they try and fail, they will be out of options and

hopeless. It is therefore better to save this option and hold out hope, even though there is no intention to enroll or invest in therapy.

- **Been There, Done That:** Through past failures in therapy, a client may become embittered to all therapy. For some, this is a defense mechanism; a protection against the fear of another failure. This type of negative attitude and inflexibility usually results in yet another failed attempt in therapy, fulfilling their belief that there is no hope and they therefore resist trying.

Other Therapeutic Profiles

The Refresher

Many clients simply need a "refresher course" using the treatment program they previously had to regain their skills. Like most programs that change behavior, without support after treatment, skills can tend to diminish over time. Clinicians need to be versed in many fluency techniques to be able to substantially replicate the critical elements of a program that had been successful for a client.

There usually is value in resurrecting the components of previous therapy that has been successful in the past. If the client had developed effective techniques, that is important information in understanding the nature of his experience in therapy and determining how to support his efforts in the future.

The Failure

Some clients who had attained fluency previously harbor strong feelings of failure when their skills diminish and their stuttering returns, sometimes even stronger than before. Their investment of time and money now appears to be squandered and they have lost something that was important to them. Regaining fluency is usually within fairly easy reach; however, the path to reinstating it now eludes them. This client usually needs additional counseling to become better prepared for relapse in the future.

The Disgruntled

An irritated client has little prospect of making any further gains in therapy and usually is quite vocal about not wishing to seek further treatment. Unlike "The Failure" who blames himself for having failed, "The Disgruntled" feels that an injustice has been done and that he has been wronged. Until he is able to see beyond his anger, there is little any clinician can do to assist him. Treating this type of client, the roles and expectations of the client and clinician should be clearly defined at the outset of therapy. Clients should be cautioned that little change can be expected when there is a mindset of failure. A trial period of therapy is often offered to afford a client the opportunity to demonstrate change, and one hopes he can allow himself to get far enough past his feelings to work productively on his stuttering.

Sincerely Searching

Inside, all people who stutter are seeking relief from their suffering. The vast majority of people who have been in therapy before are looking to make another attempt to overcome their stuttering. There likely have been important components of their treatment that were not included or were incomplete in previous therapies. These often involve overcoming the client's feelings and emotions related to their stuttering. In other instances, the answer the person sought was not available.

Where to Start

Clinicians might be well advised to explore with clients the successful and unsuccessful (or incomplete) components of previous therapies. Learning what worked (and what didn't work) and why, may make the current therapy attempt more effective and more efficient.

At the conclusion of the first session, the clinician should map out a course of action for the next month, to be used as a trial. This should include a straightforward explanation of the clinician's opinion of the client's prognosis based on assessment of their attitude, residual skills, and responsiveness to therapy techniques during the initial session. The parameters of the changes needing to be achieved by the client should be made explicitly clear. The clinician needs to demonstrate an attitude of optimism, blended with realism. Failures in previous therapy need not be a negative prognostic indicator of future success.

Consumers of Our Services

What can we learn from people who have had stuttering therapy? To learn about their experiences, McClure and Yaruss (2003) surveyed members of the National Stuttering Association who had sought help to overcome their stuttering. Their study revealed that 85% of those responding to the survey had had two or more experiences in different treatment programs or different types of treatment, and 31% had made five or more attempts to overcome their stuttering. A wide variety of approaches were reported, but none was reported to be as effective as speech therapy. Other methods included physical and mental approaches. Physical treatments included assistive devices, medications, herbal cures, electroshock, acupuncture, chiropractic therapy, and tongue surgery. The authors reported mental approaches to include hypnosis, psychiatry, motivational courses, and consulting faith healers.

Of those who received speech therapy (Table 1–1), respondents found attempts to help them change their attitude about stuttering to have been the most helpful approach. Clients also felt therapy was effective in enabling them to better manage their stuttering moments, but experienced the least success in being able to reliably manage fluent speech.

In terms of the impact of their stuttering, 80% revealed that their stuttering diminished or impeded their job performance, and 40% reported having been denied a job or

Table 1-1. Consumer Satisfaction with Stuttering Therapy

Treatment Approach	Very Successful	Somewhat Successful	Not at All Successful
Changing Attitudes Toward Speaking and Stuttering	50%	39%	10%
Learning Ways to Stutter More Easily	30%	57%	13%
Learning Ways to Speak so as Not to Stutter	19%	53%	27%

Source: Data from McClure and Yaruss (2003).

promotion as a result of their speech. Many (69%) were embarrassed by their stuttering and 81% avoided speaking situations as a result. Just over two thirds found stuttering to interfere with their family and social life.

Families of children who stutter often have too little knowledge of stuttering and no prior experience with speech therapy. Most are honestly concerned about their disfluent child and what the future holds for him. Parents are supposed to be his children's guardian and protector, but stuttering represents a domain in which they are ill-equipped to fulfill this parental role. Consequently, the speech pathologist plays a critical function in supporting parents and serving the needs of the child.

Because there is a hereditary component to stuttering, some parents may themselves be familiar with the effects of stuttering; some may have had therapy (successful or unsuccessful) before. A good deal has likely changed since the parent's therapy experience and it may be important to discuss that with concerned parents. Often, the stuttering parent projects his or her experience stuttering into their child's future. The concerns of these parent's can seem somehow more urgent.

It is important to understand the mindset of people seeking our services and the experiences they have had before coming to us. The clinician needs to be both optimistic and realistic in communicating what therapy can do for potential clients. There are several components of this message that are important to convey. For young children, research shows that nearly 80% recover from their stuttering. Rather than "wait and see," parents can be shown how to contribute by managing the child's environment to facilitate the process. For adults, stuttering therapy cannot cure stuttering, but it can provide a means of managing it effectively. The clinician can show the client the way, but cannot do the work herself. The client is responsible for making changes, for managing his speech fluency, and for setting the pace of his progress. An experienced clinician can identify the signs, symptoms, and behaviors that impact a client's prognosis for improvement. However, each client is a unique individual and caution must be taken not to imply that the results others have experienced will also be found for every other client.

In the chapters that follow, the role of the clinician and the tools used in therapy are discussed. Stuttering therapy is both an art and a science. The science (what we know and understand about stuttering) continues to emerge. The art (how we apply what we know about stuttering and what we know about people who stutter) is the hope for those who stutter. Stuttering therapy is a professional challenge for the clinician and a personal challenge for each person who stutters.

References

Ham, R. (1999). *Clinical management of stuttering in older children and adults.* Gaithersburg, MD: Aspen Publications.

Luterman, D. M. (2008). *Counseling persons with communication disorders and their families.* Austin, TX: Pro-Ed.

McClure, J. A., & Yaruss, J. S. (2003, May 13). Stuttering survey suggests success of attitude-changing treatment. *ASHA Leader.* Accessed 6/9/11 from http://www.asha.org/Publications/leader/2003/030513/030513e.htm

CHAPTER

2

Childhood Stuttering

There are significant differences between the orientation toward managing children who stutter and the ways we work with adolescent and adult clients. Children have a good chance of recovering from stuttering, whereas with adults the outcome goal is learning to manage their stuttering effectively. Therefore, information on childhood stuttering and stuttering in adolescents and adults has been separated into two chapters.

With children in the early stages of stuttering we are cautious not to bring their disfluencies to their awareness or attach any negative values to them as this appears to be one of the factors leading to the progression of stuttering to more pronounced levels. As a consequence, our work comes in manipulating variables in the child's environment and supporting his development in any delays in any function or skills that underlie speaking. An additional strategy is to reinforce their seemingly innate ability to speak more "smoothly" because it pleases others, and makes them happy.

Some children coming to us for therapy have already developed beyond simple, effortless repetitions and are aware of the difficulties they have speaking. It is still possible for these children to recover, but at this point they also need more direct intervention using speaking strategies that help them manage the stuttering that has already emerged. This chapter presents information for both groups of children and offers suggestions in working with their parents.

Chapter Outline

An Overview of Childhood Stuttering

Although the precise cause of stuttering has not yet been determined, there is reason to believe that children who stutter are born with a predisposition to do so. This constitutional vulnerability results in children's speech becoming disfluent when certain factors place strains on components of the speech system. When the stressors exceed the child's speaking capability, the flow of speech is disrupted, creating speech disfluencies or stuttering.

It is thought that this predisposition is inherited in about half of children who stutter. In others, their unique genetic makeup may render one or more components of their speech system vulnerable to disruption. The factors that stress the speech system arise from at least two sources: the development of skills and abilities that underlie speech and the factors present in the child's environment. Stuttering results when these factors strain the child's speaking system beyond its functional capacity (Starkweather, 1987).

Developmental Factors

Childhood is a period when physical, cognitive, emotional, social, and linguistic skills undergo exceptional periods of growth. Typically, the rate of growth across these domains is uneven. Growth spurts are commonly noted in one or more domains throughout childhood. Thus, it is natural for growth in one area to outpace growth in other areas throughout a child's development. For example, it is not uncommon for a child to experience rapid growth in physical dimensions, whereas growth of language skills may seemingly be at a standstill by comparison. When growth in one area outpaces growth in other areas, there is a developmental imbalance. But, typically, development in the other areas "catches up," enabling equal function across the domains. Learning a foreign language as an adult may serve as an example. At an early stage in the learning process, comprehension skills in the new language exceed expressive ability; you can understand more in the new language than you can speak. But with time, the expressive skills and the comprehension skills even out and you become able to speak as well as you can comprehend what is being spoken to you. For the child who stutters, however, during these periods of unequal development, an imbalance can occur in which a child's abilities in one domain exceed his capabilities in other areas. These lesser developed areas can become flooded by the demands placed on them by the more developed areas. For example, when a child's development in the cognitive domain exceeds his language development, he may know things about his environment but is unable to express them because his linguistic skills have not yet developed sufficiently to match his cognitive ability. Thus, he knows things, but has not developed a vocabulary or communication tools to express them. In situations such as this, the child's facility to communicate fluently may be inadequate, and speech disfluencies result. But, as his language skills catch up to his cognitive development, his speech fluency returns. This could explain why stuttering is commonly observed to "come and go" over time; the variability reflects the relative differences in developmental growth across all the domains of development and is reflected in their speech fluency.

Some children may be born with imperfect physical structures or a diminished ability to move and coordinate them, especially for speaking. In these instances, the mechanism lacks sufficient capability to speak fluently, particularly as demands for speaking more quickly increase. Some children who stutter have additional impairments, such as apraxia or motor-speech problems, which can additionally affect their speech and stuttering.

Environmental Factors

A child's communicative environments can also serve to disrupt speech fluency by pressuring the speaking system beyond its capability. Stresses can include a very busy lifestyle, family emergencies, instability in the home, rapid speaking style of other family members, use of an adult vocabulary or complex sentence structure, inattentive listeners, competition for speaking time, or even the manner in which questions are asked. These demands tend to hurry the child and cause him to try to function beyond his capability. As a consequence of these environmental pressures, stuttering results.

It is important to remember that neither developmental nor environmental factors are the cause of stuttering; they merely serve to precipitate it. In summary, it is believed that children who stutter have a speech system that is constitutionally vulnerable to disruption by developmental and environmental factors, which often interact in complex ways to disrupt a child's ability to produce smooth flowing speech. It is important for clinicians to adopt a philosophy of stuttering upon which to base treatment and to communicate effectively with parents and other related professionals, such as the child's teacher.

Developmental Levels of Stuttering

Stuttering often develops into progressively more pronounced forms. In Table 2–1, Guitar (2006) categorizes levels of stuttering in terms of speech characteristics, secondary behaviors, and the child's reactions to his speech disfluencies. A significant factor in the development of stuttering appears to be the child's awareness (and concern) about his speaking ability. As a result, special precautions should be taken *not* to draw undue attention or alarm to the child's speech in the early stages of this disorder. Children are very perceptive and sensitive to their parent's reaction to their speech and sometimes they have already become attuned to their concerns by the time they come to see a speech pathologist. Again, the parental concern is not the cause of stuttering, but can contribute to its development; in most instances, stuttering is an underlying physiologic condition.

Even though a child may become aware of his disfluencies and exhibit some distress, therapy can still be effective in promoting the return of normal, natural speech fluency. However, children's awareness and degree of concern are critical factors in enabling them to manage their speech fluency effectively. But as stuttering progresses into the intermediate and advanced stages, the goal for the outcome of therapy changes from attaining *normal fluency* to learning to manage *controlled fluency*.

Table 2–1. Characteristics of Developmental Levels of Stuttering

Developmental Level	Speech Characteristics	Secondary Behaviors	Feelings and Attitudes
Normal Disfluency	• 10 or fewer disfluencies/100 words • Single-unit repetitions • Mostly repetitions, interjections, and revisions	• None	• Unaware, no concern
Borderline Stuttering	• 11 or more disfluencies/100 words • More than 2 units of repetition • More repetitions and prolongations than revisions or interjections	• None	• Generally not aware • May occasionally show momentary surprise or mild frustration
Beginning Stuttering	• Rapid, irregular, tense repetitions • May have fixed articulatory positions in blocks	• Escape behaviors (i.e., eye blinks, increase in pitch or loudness as disfluency progresses)	• Aware of disfluency • May express frustration
Intermediate Stuttering	• Blocks in which sound and airflow are stopped	• Escape and avoidance behaviors	• Fear, frustration, embarrassment, and shame
Advanced Stuttering	• Long tense blocks	• Escape and avoidance behaviors	• Fear, frustration, embarrassment, and shame • Negative self-concept

Source: Reprinted with permission from Wolters Kluwer (2006) from B. Guitar, *Stuttering: An Integrated Approach to Its Nature and Treatment* (3rd ed., p. 167).

Pertinent Facts About Stuttering

We continue to learn more and more about stuttering from research. Parents with concerns about stuttering usually are very interested in learning more about the disorder. Too often, parents find questionable or misleading information about stuttering on the Internet. The clinician can play an important role in providing and guiding parents through what is known (and not known) about stuttering. Yairi and Ambrose (2005) offer these facts as they relate to children who stutter.

- **The Onset of Stuttering.** About 80% of children who show signs of stuttering go on to recover. Recovery usually takes more than 1 year, and sometimes as long as

5 years. A large percentage of children recover within 3 years of onset. Children who begin to stutter at a younger age appear more likely to recover.

- **Severity of Stuttering Symptoms.** The frequency (severity) of stuttering behaviors does not appear to be a predictor of recovery. However, children who do recover show a decrease in stuttering frequency over the first year following onset; children whose frequency remains the same or increases during the first year appear to be more prone to have their stuttering persist.
- **Gender.** About four or five times as many males stutter as females. Males also are at a greater risk of their stuttering persisting. Of children who eventually recover, girls seem to recover more often and faster.

Clinical Observation: An equal number of males and females stutter in early childhood, but females are more likely to recover. The gender ratio is nearly 1:1 (males to females) in early childhood, but becomes 5:1 by adulthood. However it is often observed clinically that females whose stuttering persists tend to be more resistant to speech therapy.

- **Heredity.** Stuttering often is observed to run in families. Children who have a relative who recovered from stuttering are more likely to recover themselves. Thus, those with relatives whose stuttering persisted appear to have a greater likelihood of their stuttering persisting. This likely is the most powerful prognostic factor in determining if the child's stuttering will continue or if he will recover.
- **Secondary Characteristics.** Children who do not show a decline in reactions to their stuttering (such as facial grimaces or head and neck movements) within the first year after onset of their stuttering are more prone to have their stuttering persist.
- **Articulation Skills.** In the first year after onset, children who show poorer accuracy in making sounds used in speech have a greater likelihood of their stuttering becoming chronic.
- **Other.** Stuttering is not an emotional problem, yet many children react to their stuttering in emotional ways. Stuttering is not the result of poor parenting; however, parenting styles and communication interaction styles can influence the frequency of stuttering.

This information stems from observations of many children who stutter. The researchers (Yairi & Ambrose, 2005) noted that there was great variability among the performances of the children they studied. As a consequence, this information should be used as a guideline, not an absolute predictive tool to determine the persistence of or recovery from stuttering.

Adults who stutter have been studied using PET scans (positive emission tomography) and fMRI (functional magnetic resonance imaging). Results of these studies reveal that adults who stutter use their brain in different ways when they stutter (DeNil et al., 2003). Essentially, for fluent speakers, the left hemisphere of the brain serves to coordinate activity in both hemispheres for the purpose of speaking. In those who stutter, brain activity appears present more equally distributed between both hemispheres, indicating that one side of the brain does not take a dominant or coordinating role in speaking. However, when a person who stutters speaks fluently, his brain activity is much more like that of a nonstuttering speaker. It might be inferred that the difference lies in how the brain functions, rather than the presence of a brain abnormality. Furthermore, after successful speech therapy, the brain activity among speakers who stutter had changed to be more like that of nonstuttering speakers. These results give reason for optimism as the brain of adults who stutter appears to have the capability of acquiring more normal function for speaking. Similar studies have not been completed with children due to the nature and potential risks of the neurologic testing.

Components of Evaluation and Treatment

There are several important components to include in an evaluation of the child who stutters. As treatment approaches for stuttering can include remediation for elements of a child's development, testing for delayed communication skills such as articulation, language, or cognitive skills are commonly included. Goals of the assessment may include consideration of many factors and incorporate the following:

- The child's development in the cognitive, physical, emotional, social, speech, and language domains
- An understanding of the complexities of the various environments in which the child interacts with others
- Observing the speech characteristics, secondary behaviors, and reactions to the child's speech in multiple settings to determine the developmental level of stuttering
- Determining whether the disfluencies are stuttering or normal disfluencies
- Evaluating the child's prognosis for improvement
- Determining a course of action.

The course of action selected is dependent on the child's developmental level of stuttering, his overall development, and the characteristics of the environments in which the child interacts. Generally, treatment options are based on the developmental level of stuttering. The following treatment approaches are among the most commonly pursued.

Normal Disfluencies

Client Profile

Mike's parents felt that there were more disfluencies in his speech than other children his same age. His disfluencies were single iterations of syllables and Mike wasn't even aware of them. His parents noted that there were days when he didn't have any disfluencies, but at its most pronounced there were between 7 to 9 disfluencies per 100 words. Mike, age 4, seemed to be behind his peers being able to make some of his sounds, but he talked a lot.

Treatment Approach

The clinician teaches environmental modifications to be used by the family in the home environment and communicated to participants in the child's other communicative environments. Parents are educated in modeling communicative interactions styles and advised of signs that stuttering may be emerging. A recheck typically is scheduled in three to six months.

Borderline and Beginning Stuttering

Client Profile

Jessica has had more than 12 disfluencies per 100 words for about the last 4 months. Sometimes she gets a little frustrated not being able to get some sounds out easily. Her uncle has stuttered most of his life, but not her dad. Recently she has begun to try to "push her words out." Her parents are very active and Jessica has piano lessons, soccer, and dance lessons most days after school. She's a good student but tends not to talk much in her class lately. There are times when she speaks without any disfluency, like when she plays with her dolls.

Treatment Approach

The child and parent are enrolled in treatment for a relatively small number of sessions (often six) in which environmental modifications are taught and modeled, and a system to monitor the child's daily performance is constructed. Additional client-specific information about stuttering is provided. The clinician will contact the parent to check on progress in 3 months. If the fluency hasn't improved, the child will likely be enrolled in therapy utilizing a more direct approach to modifying disfluent moments.

Intermediate and Advanced Stuttering

Client Profile

Mr. Adams has stuttered since childhood. He had therapy in school and for a short time just after starting his first job. He is very concerned about his son, Marty, who has had disfluent speech for more than a year. Marty has blocks on words beginning with plosive sounds that last a few seconds. His speech is hurried and he seems nervous when speaking to strangers and his teacher; this dramatically increases the number of blocks. Marty is very embarrassed and angry about his speech.

Treatment Approach

The child is enrolled in weekly individual therapy sessions with home practice and assignments. Group therapy and support groups (often for the parents) also may be recommended. Therapy is individually designed to address the specific needs unique to each client. Speech targets will be selected to enable the child to modify his stuttering and speak in ways more compatible with fluency. Some of the feelings and emotions about stuttering should be included in sessions. Therapy progresses at the pace of the child; therefore, the duration of therapy depends on many factors that can be difficult to predict.

Characteristics of Childhood Stuttering

One of the more difficult decisions speech pathologists are called on make is determining if a child is stuttering or if his disfluencies are typical of periods that most children go through, then, deciding what course of action should be taken. Much is written about making this decision based on the type and frequency of disfluencies, how long they have persisted, whether the child has become aware of them, and the variability of the disfluencies over time. In many cases, knowing with absolute certainty whether the child is stuttering or not can be a difficult determination to make, especially at the borderline level (Guitar, 2006). However, the course of action prescribed, whether there is stuttering or not, may not be such a difficult decision. A child who is disfluent (but not stuttering) may also need help. The presence of so many disfluencies may be reason for concern, even though they may not be considered stuttering. A case might easily be made that this child could benefit from therapy too, even though stuttering is not the diagnosis. The clinician needs to exercise ethical discretion in diagnosing stuttering if it cannot be supported from the data collected after evaluating the child. Adhering to the guidelines of "customary practice" in making any diagnosis is the most prudent course for speech pathologists to follow.

Stuttering is composed of different types of disfluencies in a child's speech. The most common are repetitions, prolongations, and blocks. Stuttering usually begins with easy, almost effortless repetitions of initial sounds or syllables at the beginning of utterances. Instances of the onset of stuttering beginning with blocks is less common, but nonetheless have been reported. The frequency of the disfluencies is important as a measure of how often in the speaking process the system breaks down. We are aware that the physical environment and emotion state in which the child is speaking may also influence his fluency. It is important to observe the child's speech in both a calm, relaxed surrounding and under conditions of greater excitement. Ten or fewer disfluencies per 100 words is considered to be "normal" and not of concern.

Clients (of any age) who are aware of their stuttering may try their best to hide it from others. Some are on guard to such a degree that they do not show any disfluencies, especially with strangers. However, there usually are signs, such as frequent pausing, interjections, word switching, loss of eye contact, or other "tells" which belie their ploy. Still others elect not to speak much under these circumstances.

Guitar's (2006) categorization of speech behaviors is very helpful in classifying the child's level of stuttering (see Table 2–1). The levels are based on the type of disfluencies, presence of secondary characteristics, and the child's awareness of and reaction to them. Note that the prominent feature in distinguishing between "stuttering" and "not stuttering" (Guitar's Normal and Borderline categories) is the element of the child's awareness. The presence of secondary characteristics is an important determinant in establishing the diagnosis of stuttering. However, neither the presence of secondary characteristics nor even blockages indicate that the client's prognosis for recovery is poor. Even children with notable blocks and secondary behaviors have recovered.

Although stuttering frequently includes repetitions, clinicians should attend to the unit that is being repeated; whether it is a sound, syllable, single-syllable word, multiple-syllable word, or a short phrase (Table 2–2). Generally, repetition of sounds and syllables are characteristic of stuttered disfluencies. But, again, there is some overlap between stuttering and normal disfluency in instances of single-syllable word repetitions. The number of times the unit is repeated is also a critical factor. Repetitions of multiple-syllable words and short phrases (and sometimes single-syllable words) are more characteristic of individuals who do not stutter.

Also of interest is the number of iterations of repetition a unit is repeated. In the disfluency "ba-ba-ba-baseball," the syllable "ba" is repeated three times. It is uttered once, and then repeated three more times. Generally speaking, the more iterations, the more likely the disfluency is considered to be stuttered. Two or more iterations of repetition are considered to be more typical of stuttering.

Table 2–2. Classification of Repetitions*

Type of Repetition	Example	Classification
Single-sound	S-s-s-softball	Likely stuttering if more the two iterations of repetition
Single-syllable word	Ba-ba-ba-baseball	Likely stuttering if more than two iterations of repetition
Part-word	Mini-mini-minimum	Less typical of stuttering, but in question
Whole-word	Marie, Marie, Marie is my friend.	Less typical of stuttering
Phrase	The big horse. the big horse jumped really high.	Less typical of stuttering

*Overlap exists between categories. For example, the word "I" is both a single sound and a whole word. Look for the frequency of occurrence in the overall speech sample to help determine whether repetitions are stuttering or typical of normal disfluencies. The unit being repeated, the number of iterations of repetition, and the overall number of repetitions per 100 words contribute to distinguishing between stuttering and normal disfluencies.

Escape behaviors are the client's attempts to free himself from his stuttering. They are considered secondary behaviors because they are the child's reactions to his disfluencies. Escape behaviors occur *after* a disfluency has begun. Escape behaviors commonly include blinking the eyes, head jerks, facial grimaces, or increased struggle behavior (as indicated by visible muscle tension), rising pitch, or increasing the intensity (loudness) of speech. Escape behaviors are indicative of the child's increased muscle tension and struggle.

Client Profile

Each time Daniel had a stuttering block, even a mild one, his head bobbed a little as if to shake the word out of his mouth. After a few weeks, the head bobbing seemed to become a permanent feature of his stuttering, but now his volume got louder and louder as he tried to push words out. This seemed to work intermittently, helping him to get through difficult words. It wasn't long before it no longer was effective, but Daniel kept doing it nonetheless. The only thing it did was to make his stuttering look more severe.

Another behavior is avoidance or the client's attempt not to stutter when he feels a disfluency to be eminent. Rather than stutter, the child may pause or switch words for ones he is confident that he can say. Frequent hesitations while speaking or pauses in unlikely places when uttering sentences likely are avoidance behaviors. Even though the disfluency has not surfaced, we can infer that an instance of stuttering has taken (or would have taken) place; the child has not let it happen by his attempts to avoid it. Successfully avoiding disfluencies is not the same as fluency because what was intended to be communicated was disrupted by the fear of stuttering. Over time, avoidance behaviors gain strength and serve to increase the client's fears of stuttering. When faced with the belief that he will stutter, the client has choices: to proceed and perhaps stutter, or to avoid the feared word. When the choice is to proceed, the likely outcome will be to stutter, as experienced in many past instances. When the fear of stuttering is evoked, clients often and unconsciously respond with tension in the muscles that move the structures and use more force in trying to articulate the sound or word. When the choice is to avoid the word, the client has submitted to his fears. As a consequence, the fear becomes stronger and the next instance in which the word appears, the choice more likely will be to avoid it again as the fear this time is greater. Before long, it is no longer a conscious choice because the child feels that saying the word is impossible.

Next, the fear can be generalized to other words that begin with the same sound or to other situations in which stuttering has occurred in the past. As fears grow in intensity and are encountered more frequently, some children opt to talk less and less, effectively shutting down expressive communication. This is not uncommon among children coming to a "strange place" for their speech to be evaluated. Consequently, it is important to gather information about the child's willingness to interact and speak in other communication situations such as in the classroom, playing with friends, social gatherings with relatives, and the like. This information helps to paint a broader picture of the impact or handicap of the child's stuttering.

Evaluating Stuttering in Children

An evaluation of a child who is disfluent includes a variety of components based upon the needs of the child, parent, and clinician. Common objectives in evaluating children who stutter include: (a) establishing a diagnosis (often distinguishing between stuttering and normal disfluencies), (b) assessing the development of speaking-related system components, (c) collecting information about the child's communication environments, (d) documenting the current status of the child's communication skills, (e) establishing a prognosis, and (f) determining a course of action. These objectives are accomplished through formal and informal testing, observation, and information gathering from the parent.

History

We are interested in gathering information about the onset of the stuttering and the course of its development to the present time. Information about the child's general development enables us to glean insights into the growth of the various speech-related domains discussed earlier. Also of interest is whether other family members stutter and the course and progression of their stuttering. Information about the child's environment is a topic of significance (the pace of communication interactions in the home, situations with child care, siblings, parental interaction styles, etc.). Getting a picture of the home and other communication environments helps paint the picture of the world in which the child needs to be able to communicate and the stresses he may place upon him. The case history interview also can be helpful in learning about other conditions the child may have, his temperament, and socialization skills. Of additional importance is determining the parent's level of the concern about the child's speech.

Clinical Insight: Providing therapy for children, there are two customers to serve—the child and the parent. As speech pathologists, we focus on aspects of the client's communication difficulties and the factors that underlie it. We keep an eye open for how we will treat the client and develop the most appropriate and effective treatment plan. Frequently, parents are additionally concerned about broader issues, such as their child not having friends, his ability to compete verbally in the classroom, or his potential of getting a good job in the future. It therefore is critically important to allow the parents opportunities to express their apprehensions so that we are sure to address their concerns as well as our own. Savvy clinicians enhance customer satisfaction when they treat the client's stuttering and also respond to parental worries.

Stuttering

The assessment of the child's disfluencies is the main purpose of the evaluation and is the component examined most completely. Important elements include descriptions of the types, duration, and frequency of disfluencies observed. This information also aids the clinician in distinguishing between normal and stuttered disfluencies and yields a measure of overt stuttering severity. A purpose of the evaluation is to observe the child in a calm, relaxed surrounding and under conditions of excitement that are likely increase the frequency of stuttering symptoms. Secondary characteristics are also noted. The presence of secondary characteristics implies that the child is aware of his speech difficulties, because we consider secondary characteristics to be a child's reaction to his stuttering. To react, the child must be aware. However, this should not be interpreted as giving the clinician license to talk about the disfluencies openly.

Assessing the child's awareness of stuttering is a delicate proposition. Recall that we do not wish to draw inappropriate or unfavorable attention to the child's disfluencies. Consequently, care should be taken to broach talk of the disfluencies in a delicate manner. One approach is to refer to them using nonpejorative terms, such as "bumps," instead of using labels for the disfluencies, like calling them "stuttering." The terminology can facilitate a discussion about the client's speech without attaching any negative inferences. The clinician reflects an attitude about the client's "bumps" such that bumps aren't bad, but smooth speech is preferable. Analogously, a person might express that vanilla ice cream isn't bad, but she just prefers chocolate.

It is important to determine if there are specific sounds, words, or circumstances in which the stuttering is more prominent. Some clients who stutter have more difficulty on sounds that require finer motor coordination or, often, plosive sounds in which the nature of their production entails building up intraoral breath pressure, which in a way feels like the beginnings of having a stuttering block.

A discussion can reveal not only the child's awareness of his disfluencies, but also his level of concern about them. Again, the clinician's posture is not to imply that disfluencies are in any way bad or that anything is wrong, but only to demonstrate her interest in learning more about them. The child's awareness and feelings about his stuttering need also to be included in the calculation of the rating of the severity of stuttering.

Many children are already aware of their stuttering and have begun to react to it emotionally. These children may be looking for help and it is healthy for the child to have an avenue available to him to talk about his stuttering openly and objectively. Stuttering should be discussed in objective (rather than emotional) terms, respectful of the child as an otherwise intact, likable person. Feeling alone with a stuttering problem can turn the child inward in looking for a source of blame for his speech. Being able to talk about stuttering with others in his environment, his parents, teachers, and speech pathologist, goes a long way in supporting the child.

Other Parameters of Communication

Children who stutter have been found to have a higher incidence of articulation and language problems than the general population. Consequently, we need to screen the other parameters of communication (articulation, language development, voice, and hearing) that may complicate our treatment of stuttering or necessitate treatment of these problems concurrently. When the child does not pass the screening in any of these areas, an in-depth evaluation should be forthcoming prior to initiating treatment. Many formal or informal screening procedures are available to the clinician.

Affect and Personality Traits

Like all children, those who stutter vary in terms of their personality. Some children (including those who stutter) are more shy and reticent than others, as seen in their reluctance to separate from parents or interact with unfamiliar persons. Their apparent apprehension in new surroundings and with new people likely decreases their willingness to interact or speak. We understand that under these conditions their speech is likely to contain more disfluencies than is typical. However, it is unclear whether children who stutter are more sensitive than children who do not, and therefore more likely to stutter.

Shyness is not always characteristic of children who stutter, even though a subset of children who stutter would be considered shy or withdrawn. What is of interest is the child's willingness to communicate with others. Many children who stutter are very outgoing verbally and do not seem to let their disfluencies get in their way. Shy or outgoing, the clinician needs to observe the child's willingness to interact with others as a measure of communication effectiveness or the severity their difficulties represent.

Motor Skills

Speech is a motor act and motor skills and motor coordination develop throughout childhood. It is of interest to inquire as to the child's general motor development through his achievement of common motor milestones and fine motor activities such as eating, chewing, drooling, and swallowing. Another indicator of motor ability is the development of articulation skills and sound mastery milestones. Children with difficulty mastering fine motor skills or midline movements that have not resolved may present reason for concern over the integrity of oral-motor skills as it impacts fluency. A gross assessment of current oral motor function can be obtained by testing the child's diadochokenetic ability. Children with apraxia, dysarthria, or neuromuscular impairments are also known to stutter.

Case Examples

Let's contrast two children who began to stutter, comparing their speech characteristics, development, home environment and the course of action that was taken in each case.

Client Profile: Mark

Unlike his older sister, Mark began putting words together a little behind developmental norms. His parents were concerned about his speaking ability too at that point; his speech seemed a little labored and his disfluencies were very apparent. In sharp contrast, Mark was early to walk and he seemed to be constantly on the move. Mark's dad had stuttered as a child, but he had "outgrown it" in childhood. That made his father all the more concerned about Mark's speech.

The family was very active and Mark and his sister were always going somewhere in the family van—skating, dance lessons, picnicking, play groups, grocery shopping, and the like. Even at home, it seemed that there was always something going on for Mark—kicking the ball with dad outside, making block castles, playing hide and seek. While one parent entertained the children, the other was usually engaged in some sort of chore around the house. Like many households, Mark's was sometimes a little chaotic. Sometimes the children seemed to need to compete to get parental attention. At busier times, this seemed to be reflected in the fluency of Mark's speech. The parents had been concerned about Mark's speech for about a year. In the beginning, his disfluencies were mostly syllable repetitions; although he was beginning to struggle a little now to get words out, it seemed that overall, there were fewer disfluencies in his speech now than when they had started.

Factor Analysis

Concerns—This child appears to be delayed in his development of speech and language skills. The family's lifestyle is active and there is competition for talking time within the family unit. Because of his own stuttering, Mark's father may be reacting to his son's disfluencies without recognizing it.

Positive Indicators—Mark's disfluencies began at an early age and even though he showed signs of struggle, the frequency of his disfluencies decreased with time. Yairi and Ambrose (2005) found that children who began to stutter still recovered after stuttering for up to 48 months. They also found that the presence of struggle behaviors was not a predictor of persistent stuttering. In this case we also note a family history of recovery from stuttering.

Course of Action—Mark's parents were concerned enough to seek help. The speech pathologist worked to help Mark develop language and articulation skills and offered the parents suggestions about reducing the pace and competitiveness for talking at home, which they were quick to implement. We are happy to report that, 8 months later, Mark's speech disfluencies had all but disappeared, but the family continued to modify their interaction style in the home.

Client Profile: Haley

Haley was an only child and her development followed milestones pretty closely. At about 4 years of age, just as she began preschool, her mother noticed that Haley was starting to struggle making some sounds when talking. Haley's grandfather had a mild stuttering problem that persisted throughout his life. A single mom, Haley's mother works two jobs to meet ends meet. Haley likes her babysitter in the afternoons after preschool and they get along well. The household has a fairly relaxed atmosphere. Haley is well behaved, a bit reserved, and likes to read books and often plays by herself with her toys. Over the past year, Haley's disfluencies have waxed and waned, but overall their frequency has not decreased. Although she doesn't seem bothered by them, other children are beginning to notice them, as has the preschool teacher. Haley's mom is reluctant to take time off from work to have her tested. Starting school next year, she will be sure that Haley gets screened by the speech therapist, and if therapy is needed, she will be able to get it at school.

When school started, Haley was seen by the speech therapist. However, she didn't notice any disfluencies as Haley didn't talk much during the screening. As a consequence, no services were recommended. At the present time, Haley still is quite disfluent, especially when she visits her dad. On visitation days, her disfluencies were always more pronounced and struggle behaviors began to emerge.

Factor Analysis

Concerns—Haley's stuttering started later than is the average. Yairi and Ambrose (2005) reported that 70% of cases experience the onset of stuttering by at 42 months. There also is a family history of persistent stuttering. Haley's stuttering has not decreased in frequency over the first year. As previously mentioned, although there still remains plenty of time for her stuttering to resolve, but the fact that the frequency of disfluency has not decreased is worrisome. Her shy temperament is felt by some to increase her risk for stuttering.

Positive Indicators—Statistically, her gender is in Haley's favor in terms of potentially recovering. Her physical and language development appear to be normal. Her home environment likely provides security, but the stresses at her school and with the parental visitation situation appear to present problems for Haley.

Course of Action—Although her rationale was understandable, Haley appears to have fallen through the cracks as she started school. In second grade, her stuttering became much more pronounced, attracting the attention and comments of her classmates. She became much more concerned about her difficultly speaking. At this point, Haley has enrolled in therapy, but only after the problem had become more apparent.

Summary of the Case Comparisons

It is typical for the indicators to be mixed, that is, for there to be a combination of concerns and positive indications that the stuttering will resolve. Remember that the indicators that we have are statistics and provide us with information about stuttering amongst a group of children. Each child is an individual and his unique characteristics likely differ in one or more ways from the norm of the group.

From Yairi and Ambrose (2005), we find several prognostic indicators of recovery, which include the following:

- A family history of recovery from stuttering
- An early onset of stuttering
- Strong phonological and nonverbal skills
- An overall decrease in the frequency of disfluencies over the first year since onset, especially for females
- The duration of disfluencies (how long each one lasts) is *not* a negative indicator
- The overt severity of stuttering is *not* a negative prognostic sign
- A child's awareness or reactions to his or her disfluencies did *not* prove to be an indication that stuttering would persist.

Of these factors, family history was found to be the strongest predictor. Children having a relative whose stuttering persisted were more likely for their stuttering to persist. Those with a family member who recovered, were themselves more likely to recover.

Yairi and Ambrose (2005) found that approximately one-third of children they studied had a sudden onset of stuttering, whereas the remainder reported a more gradual, intermittent beginning. They also observed some stuttering begins at a more severe level of stuttering. Among their subjects, 76% developed normal fluency (recovered) within 4 years of onset, while the stuttering of 24% continued to become chronic.

As a lesson to clinicians, remember there is a great deal of variability in stuttering and what is important is the one, unique child and his family who has come to you for help.

Treatment Approaches

There are two distinct directions in treating children who stutter, depending on their awareness and concern about their disfluencies. For children who have limited or no awareness of their stuttering, an indirect approach is usually preferred. Their treatment incorporates three components; reinforcing the child's nature ability to produce "smooth speech," manipulation of environmental factors that provide communication stress, and remediation of any delays or deficiencies in speech-related domains such as articulation skills, language abilities, social and cognitive development, and oral-motor skills.

Children who are conscious of their stuttering and react to it need to develop some strategies to deal with their difficult speech. Treatment includes many of the components listed above, but more direct therapy to assist the child dealing with the speech aspects of his stuttering are involved.

Children Who Are Unaware of Their Stuttering

Due to the child's limited awareness of his disfluencies, caution is taken in discussing his speech and how people react to it. Children are well attuned to the emotional reactions of their parents as well as the words used to describe the concerns over their speech. As a consequence, consideration needs to be given to the words used to discuss the child's speech and the gestures and mannerisms displayed during the discussion, taking care not to use negative or pejorative words in reference to the child or his speech. Use caution not to display worry, exasperation, concern, or disapproval in the speaker's attitude, tone or gestures. Detaching emotions from a conversation about the concern about the child's speech is not always easy as our speech patterns often belie what we are feeling. It often is beneficial to explain this to the parent prior to an evaluation or consultation. The clinician is responsible for setting the tone and modeling an objective, neutral character for the conversations about the child, his stuttering behaviors, and the parent's concerns.

To help maintain discretion, discussion of the child's disfluencies might be broached indirectly using techniques that include partner modeling, environmental management, and remediation of development deficiencies related to communication. Therapy usually incorporates the parents extensively in the treatment protocol. The clinician works to educate them about their child's stuttering and to train them to work with the child in other settings. Parents generally spend the most time with their children, particularly preschoolers. They also have a strong vested interest in the outcome of treatment and can teach others in their child's environment about creating an optimal atmosphere for fluency. As a consequence, educating and training parents is an integral part of the success of therapy.

Modeling

Modeling is a very powerful clinician tool, particularly with children. Good storytellers enhance the listener's mental image of a story by using intonation, inflection, and varying vocal intensity in their speech. Likewise, good clinicians can use modeling to set the tone and pace of therapy. It is hard for a client to learn to speak slowly and softly when the clinician is speaking quickly and loudly. For the clinician, when it comes to teaching clients to modify their speaking style, you need to "say it and show it." All people are impacted by their speaking environment, but for the child who stutters, the results of trying to keep pace with a quick speaking partner inevitably lead to disfluency.

Preschoolers usually spend the major portion of their time in the home and other social situations with peers, such as play groups, preschool, and siblings. Communication settings outside of the treatment room are the most influential in the child's world. It is common for children who stutter to become fluent in the clinic, but be disfluent in other environments. The clinic environment usually lacks the interruptions, spontaneous interactions, and surprises that are commonplace in other situations. It takes considerable time and effort to bring fluency from the treatment room into the real world. This job typically is left primarily to the parents. Creating an optimal communication environment is often a real challenge for families, but the results are well worth the effort.

Case Example

Four-year-old Brittany has a good many repetitions at the beginning of many of her utterances; usually three or four iterations. Speaking at a slower rate seems to reduce her repetitions. In therapy, she and the clinician have a tea party. The clinician asks Brittany questions, modeling the slower speaking rate she wants her to imitate. After Brittany answers each question, the clinician echoes back Brittany's response, again using the desired slow rate.

Environmental Management

As part of the home communication environment, parents are instructed to stop what they are doing and give their child their full attention, stopping any activity and looking directly at the child in an attentive, comfortable manner. Some children feel that their message is not being heard and struggle to gain attention. Relatedly, parents, from time to time, can repeat the message that they received from the child to reassure him that he was understood. Modeling is an important component of this interaction; a slow normal rate and soft speaking voice have a calming effect, one that will optimize fluency.

Communication partners frequently ask questions, both for clarification and to stimulate more conversation. Communication pressure is sometimes relieved by asking an opinion, rather than asking for very specific factual information. For example, instead of asking, "*What is your friend at school's name?*" (a question that requires a single, specific word), the subject might be broached in a different way. It might be asked, "*You have a friend at school; what's he like?*" This second question allows the child greater latitude in responding. A specific, single word is not "the answer"; there is not a right or wrong response; it is left up to the child how to describe his friend. This subtlety lessens communication pressure, which may be reflected in the child's ability to be fluent.

Turn-taking may also be regulated within the family unit. This serves to ensure that everyone gets an uninterrupted opportunity to speak and participate. Only one person speaks at a time; everyone gets a turn. Sometimes, the speaker holds a special object designating that it is their exclusive turn to speak. When finished speaking, the object is passed to the next speaker for his turn. This reduces the pressure of trying to break into a conversation and goes a long way toward diminishing the fears of being interrupted or passed by when wishing to communicate. Again, this promotes order and discipline in the speaking environment, which lessens the stresses that might otherwise be present.

Case Example

Jimmy's family is very involved in family activities. They often go on weekend ski trips, attend his older brother's hockey games, and go to his older sister's gymnastic practices, Jimmy has band and clarinet lessons, mom takes him grocery shopping with her—they are always on the run with somewhere to go seemingly all the time. There's a lot of commotion getting into the car and making sure that everything needed is packed to go. Jimmy's speech is much more disfluent during the comings and goings. He often feels that he has to fight to get mom's or dad's attention when he tries to talk, and he rushes to speak, usually with more disfluencies. Jimmy's speech clinician suggests that everyone get a turn to speak when they are riding in the car, and that one of the parents repeat back what Jimmy has said to reassure him that his communication was successful.

Remediation of Deficiencies

It is common to find that some of a child's developmental skills or abilities are less developed than those of others the same age. In some instances, this creates an imbalance that can interfere with speaking fluently. For example, the fluency of an adult is interrupted when he is unable to recall the name of a town in time to insert it in his utterance. *"Weren't you born in _ _* (pause) *_ _ Holland?"* Or, when you become aware that you've started to say the wrong word; *"Please get another sh . . . blanket."* In a similar light, when a child begins to utter an idea, but hasn't developed a vocabulary sufficient to express his thoughts, disfluency can result. Or, a child whose oral motor coordination is underdeveloped may not be able to physically move his articulators to create the sounds that he is thinking about in his head quickly enough; disrupted speech is the outcome.

As a consequence, when associated developmental abilities are found to be delayed, therapy is often directed toward remediation and improving their function as is appropriate. This is commonly incorporated concurrently with therapy for stuttering.

Case Example

Joey has had a number of sound distortions and sound omissions as he articulated words. His development was thought to be delayed, rather than there being a physiologic problem. It seemed that he had more disfluencies on misarticulated words too. Therapy to improve Joey's articulation development was integrated into his stuttering therapy goals. The clinician worked on the two areas of his speech difficulties concurrently.

In Therapy

Initial efforts are directed toward developing fluent responses, often in the form of distinguishing between "smooth" and "bumpy" utterances. It is important not to use negative labels for features of the child's speech for fear of the child becoming more concerned or thinking he is doing something wrong or bad when he speaks. The terms "bumpy" and "smooth" are not used in a way that indicates that they are good or bad attributes. They are merely descriptions that distinguish between the two forms of speaking. The clinician or parent expresses their preference for one over the other, but neither is necessarily correct or wrong. Thus, the child is reinforced for his smooth speech and sometimes requested to remake his bumpy speech into smooth speech.

Once the child is able to manage fluency by speaking slowly and smoothly, stressors are introduced. Stressors may include the excitement of games or activities that introduce the element of excitement, speed, or motor ability in which rapid changes between gross and fine motor movement are required. These stresses simulate situations outside of therapy and attempt to challenge the child's skills managing smooth speech. Strangers can be introduced into some activities as another source of stress for the client.

Case Example

Billy's disfluencies were pretty mild and he wasn't really aware of them, or at least he didn't react to them. But, because his mother was so anxious about the possibility of them persisting, she noticeably stiffened every time he was disfluent. In therapy, the clinician calmly noted when Billy's speech was "bumpy" and asked if Billy could make it smoother as she modeled an example of how to say it smoother. He was happy to oblige because the "speech teacher" was so happy every time he "fixed" his bumpy speech.

Billy's clinician showed his mom how to do the same thing in a calm, relaxed manner, showing excitement when he smoothed his speech. The clinician also asked Billy's mother to write down the specific words Billy was disfluent on, the type of disfluency he had, and whether he was able to make it smooth at her request. Giving his mother a way to help Billy enabled her to be less anxious and stressed about his disfluent speech.

Children Who Are Aware of Their Stuttering

Many of the approaches used with children who are unaware of their stuttering can be applied to treating children who are aware of their stuttering, especially modifying environmental variables and treating concomitant problems. Additionally, the child who is concerned about his stuttering will benefit from methods of managing these disfluencies more effectively and having someone to talk with about his speech.

Similar to working with adults, the techniques (targets) used in this direct therapy are selected to address the characteristics of the child's disfluent speech that differ from normal speech production. Attention is often focused on preparing for utterances, initiating utterances, or specific words or speaking situations. The aim is to provide tools for the child to better manage his stuttering or promote greater natural fluency. Many of these techniques are similar to those used with adults, just simplified.

Get Ready to Talk

It's common that children who stutter often seem to try to talk before everything is ready to go, or that they start without a complete plan to put what they want to say into words. That, too, is seen in normally developing children. Their ability to translate an idea into words, select the right words, find the correct grammatical structure, programming to coordinate breathing, phonation, and articulation seems to still be emerging or perhaps is insufficient for the complexities of what they are trying to communicate. Add to that the perception that the speaking situation is demanding the utterance very quickly, and disfluent speech is an understandable result.

Taking one or two seconds more before beginning can remove the hurry that leads to a disjointed utterance. Building the habit of getting ready before beginning can really make a difference. It is suggested that the clinician develop a slogan or speech rule to help the child learn and heed this helpful habit. This is also helpful in combating the quickness some children demonstrate when talking and helps them get off to a good start.

Case Example

When he is in a hurry to say something, Jacob's speech sort of falls apart. It seems that he either has trouble getting started speaking or gets stuck midstream in a sentence and looks perplexed. His clinician established a speech rule: *"Don't start until you're ready."* In some ways, this gives Jacob "permission" to take more time and he doesn't feel as rushed. As a consequence, even this little bit of extra time, makes a real difference for him. When not in a hurry, he begins utterances easier and the extra time seems to be just enough for him to structure what he wants to say. Speech rules usually enhance the effectiveness of therapy with younger children who are already accustomed to having rules at home or in school.

Take a Breath

There are a couple of ways that the breath target can be used. A frequent characteristic in some children who stutter is encountering difficulty at the onset of utterances. When closer observation reveals the client is forcing his speech out, instead of initiating it gently, the breath technique may be useful. The child is instructed to take a deep breath, let about half of it out, and then begin his sentence slowly and gently. The deep breath serves to stretch and relax the muscles of respiration (his chest muscles) and the musculature in the larynx. The reduction in muscle tension better facilitates the initiation of speech. The process is further promoted by focusing on beginning the utterance gently.

The second benefit is that it assists in slowing the pace of speaking. The tendency to rush an utterance is impeded by needing to postpone starting until half of the breath has been exhaled. Being disciplined in speaking increases the client's control of the speaking process, resulting in more fluency.

Case Example

Fearful of stuttering, Timmy's tendency is to hurry his speech. He is so fearful of stuttering that he "jumps into" speaking right from the beginning of an utterance. His clinician reminds him to slow down, but he is overcome by his fear of being laughed at, and can't seem to manage it. The clinician tries a new speech rule for Timmy, "Take a Breath." He now starts out in control, by taking a deeper breath before beginning to speak. When he remembers to do it, it works great. Like any new target, taking a breath will need more practice before he can use it reliably. Timmy finds knowing what to do and being able to help himself to be very reassuring.

Easy Starts

Most stuttering occurs at the beginning of utterances. This point in the speaking process requires the most coordination and is the most complex part of producing speech. There is a split second when respiration turns from inhalation to exhalation, the vocal folds come together, and the process of articulating a long string of sounds is started, all within an extremely short period of time. When they are nervous or try to hurry the initiation of speech, children who stutter frequently seem to miscoordinate or in some other way mishandle this motor act. A common reaction seems to be to use more force in attempting to get their speech started. To help the child change this instinctive behavior, his attention is focused on slowly and gradually beginning phonation; almost like stretching the first sound, but instead of elongating the sound, it is a gradual, controlled increase in muscle tension that produces the feeling of stretching.

Case Example

Amanda seems to worry about speaking. She starts off in a hurry and it seems like she tries to "bull" her way through her speech, an extra measure just to be sure it goes well. But the result is usually a disaster and she seems to be unable to break this habit, even though it doesn't help her. Amanda's clinician suggested that she start off very softly, then get louder once she gets going; they call this an Easy Start.

Now Amanda has another approach to getting started, one that works much better for her. Her parents note that at home, she still goes back to her old habit every once in a while, but now she stops herself and uses the Easy Start instead. Amanda says, *"It's such a little thing to remember to do, but it really helps in a big way."*

Stretches

Making speaking less complex appears to improve a child's speech fluency. Speaking more slowly, slowing the initiation of speech, and speaking more softly each make speaking less complicated and are seen to improve fluency. Stretching is another example. Fluency is promoted by slowing the transitions between sounds, or stretching the sounds out. Using stretches not only slows the rate of speech, but focuses more of the child's attention toward speaking in a volitional, rather than automatic, way. Stretches are accomplished by elongating the vowel sounds in words; *"Myyyyyyyyyyyyy moooooooooom maaaaaaaaaaaaakes paaaaaancaaaaaaaaakes."* Children often think "stretchy speech" feels like they are talking like a robot; as long as that image is fun, it will promote its use in therapy.

Case Example

Christopher seems to stumble on words throughout his utterances. He speaks quickly and doesn't take the time to articulation all of the sounds as well as he might. Stretches help Christopher take more time speaking, which improves his articulation and his fluency. He enjoys playing with puppets in therapy and having them use their stretchy speech too. When Christopher's puppet gets stuck on a sound, he knows how to stretch the sound to get out of trouble.

Talking About Stuttering

Children who are aware of their stuttering usually have feelings about it. For some it makes them feel frustrated and angry; for others it's embarrassing or just makes them feel bad. These are the emotions that facilitate the child's attempts not to stutter. These attempts commonly take the form of speaking quickly and using more muscular effort to talk. Working to manage these emotions can serve to reduce the muscle tension that results, resulting in more natural fluency.

Children don't know how to deal with their stuttering by themselves. Talking about stuttering with the child helps him feel less alone and begins to build a support team to help him out. It's difficult for children to put their feelings into words, so the clinician needs to help the child find a venue to express these feelings. Sometimes, it can come in drawing a picture of his stuttering or an activity like ripping up or stomping on a piece of paper with the word stuttering written on it. Children also can give a talk about stuttering to their classmates to help them understand stuttering. This frequently reduces the amount of teasing and ridicule once the topic of stuttering comes out in the open and others understand it better.

Case Example

Matthew got so angry and frustrated when he couldn't get his words out. His teacher was becoming concerned that he might start hitting the children who laughed when Matthew was disfluent. She talked with the speech therapist at school about ways to manage Matthew's feelings about his stuttering. Together they decided that all the children in Matthew's class would give a talk about the way that people are different and how each is special. The speech clinician worked with Matthew to develop a talk about stuttering, one of the ways Matthew was different. After the classroom assignment had been completed, the speech therapist and Matthew talked about everyone's differences and learned that some differences were better than others, but everyone is different in "good" and "not so good" ways. Matthew was surprised to learn about the problems other kids had. Because his classmates now understood about Matthew's difference, there was much less to make fun of him about and they were impressed to learn that Matthew also had one brown eye and one blue eye!

Working with Parents

It is important to recognize that parents come for help because they are legitimately concerned about their child. In the vast majority of cases, parental concern is usually legitimate. However, there is variance in the nature and degree of their concerns and, thus, being a good listener will help the clinician understand how to address both the child's speech and the parent's concerns. Experience finds parents to be pretty accurate in screening disfluency behaviors; few parents are concerned over "nothing." For those who are unduly concerned, providing accurate information and reassurance is generally of great value to them.

The most difficult thing we can ask of parents is to "do nothing" or "wait and see." Parents of younger children in particular are usually willing to "leap over the tallest building" if called upon to do so. Advising parents to "wait and see" or not to be concerned about their child's speech is neither effectively using a valuable resource nor providing them a service. Giving parents an assignment can both ease their anxiety and provide additional data from other communication environments to which clinicians are not privy. Such assignments might include detailing the characteristics and frequency of disfluencies throughout the day; logging the environments in which the child was disfluent; recording video samples of the child's communications; or instructing parents in ways to modify their communication interactions with their child to promote more fluency. Aside from providing potentially important information for the clinician, the parents have a task, a role in their child's betterment, and it helps build a team to better support the child.

The importance of listening to the parents is to help them define their needs. Frequently, parental worries build on one another. Helping to sort out a laundry list of concerns can make the entirety of an issue seem less overwhelming and provide a new perspective of an obstacle that is somehow less insurmountable. Remember, children don't bring themselves to therapy. Although the child may be our client, the parent is our customer. The most successful clinicians work both to satisfy their customers and provide good service to their clients.

The concerns of parents of children who stutter commonly reflect anxiety about the child being ridiculed and being made to feel different in an undesirable way. These fears are often fueled when there is a family history of stuttering. Remember, it is a parent's job to protect their child from harm, be it of a physical or an emotional nature. Anxiety has the ability to sweep us up in our concerns, and worry often spreads those concerns to the child's future ability to get a good job, to find someone to marry, and to live a happy, productive life. It is important not to discount these concerns and to be forthright in dealing with them directly. Many anxieties and concerns are only aggravated when honest, objective information is not provided. Coping can only begin to take place once the truth of a situation is known. Providing a portrait of a realistic outcome can be accomplished by enabling parents to contact parents of other clients, becoming part of a support group, and even identifying adults who have succeeded in life despite their stuttering.

Our responsibility as therapists to educate parents about stuttering is particularly important in the overall treatment process. Historically, stuttering has been the subject of incredible misconceptions, many of which continue today. Knowing what stuttering is can be almost as important as knowing what it is not. It is not a psychological or emotional problem, although people who stutter usually have strong emotions about their stuttering. Furthermore, people who stutter often react to their stuttering in ways that denote that something is wrong or that there is something to be ashamed of. Behaviors such as avoidances, loss of eye contact, withdrawal, shyness, or anxiety lead the casual observer to conclude that these behaviors or traits are the cause of a stuttering problem, rather than a reaction to it.

It is important to form a team with parents because it is much harder for clinicians to resolve a child's stuttering without them. Teaming builds important communication links that can both educate and enable parents. It is of benefit for parents to observe and in many other ways be a part of treatment sessions. Time invested in training parents is usually time well spent to the benefit of the child. Parents learn to vary interaction styles and may be trained to do therapy activities in other communication environments; this extends the reach of therapy well beyond the treatment room.

Training Parents

Parents are necessarily a core component of the therapy. To maximize their utility, clinicians must educate them about the nature of stuttering, provide them with a model of stuttering, train them to become accurate, objective observers who can identify, monitor, and document aspects of the child's disfluencies, teach them how to modify speaking environments, and develop a support team in the child's other communication environments, such as his classroom at school.

Much of the parental angst about stuttering lies in what is not known or is misunderstood about it. This confusion only serves to breed more anxiety. Not knowing what to believe and what not to believe, parents naturally are perplexed and confused. Providing informational materials and discussing a model of stuttering helps parents better evaluate new information and formulate their own beliefs about their child's stuttering. Defining their role in the therapeutic process represents empowerment. It is a lot to ask a parent to "do nothing" and it is an ineffective use of this critical resource.

Another part of parent education is learning to identify different types of disfluencies and the frequency and duration of disfluent moments. Not surprisingly, this also serves to develop a more objective attitude toward stuttering, which results in the ability to discuss it with more emotional detachment. Parents also may be asked to identify specific sounds, words, and situations in which disfluencies occur. This information can be of value to the clinician in getting a broader picture of the child's stuttering and understanding its characteristics outside the treatment room. Focusing their attention on concrete, discrete behaviors helps to reduce parental fears and anxiety as their thoughts are being drawn to more objective aspects of the disorder.

To varying degrees, our speech rate is a reflection of or reaction to our environment. We follow the social conventions to determine how loud, how fast, and within what proximity we should speak. Additionally, our perception of the pace of the environment also affects how we speak. Family home environments can be rushed and somewhat chaotic, especially when there are several children. Families also undergo stresses such as a lost cat, a parental argument, loss of employment, sibling rivalries, and so forth. Many homes are fast paced and the rate of speech in the home reflects it. These factors are controllable to a degree, but it may best serve the child who stutters to create "relaxed zones," where there is a slower pace, softer speaking voices, more structure, and more individualized attention. Parents might create a story time or family hour. The idea is to create a speaking environment similar to that of the therapy room, but in the home with family members. This requires a good deal of discipline and effort to establish on the part of the parents. However, the effort can be critical to the transfer and carryover of fledgling fluency skills. Families might set up a story hour or game time in which everyone can unwind, relax and create a calm environment for interacting. Parents need to model responses and coax others who interact with their child during his day to follow suit.

Obstacles

Parental Attitudes

Although most parents are eager to become a part of the treatment team, there are those who seemingly bring their child to the clinic to be "fixed" in therapy. Their perception appears to be that their role and responsibility is to transport the child to the session and pay for it; and our responsibility is to repair the child's speech. This type parent typically spends his or her time making phone calls in the waiting room, or even leaving the clinic to run a few errands while the session is in progress. From the start, it is important to communicate and construct a role for a parent that obviates the need for their participation, right from the initial evaluation. Desired roles for parents include observing, collecting data, managing and manipulating the child's environment, modeling responses, providing feedback, advocating for the child, and leading activities and practice sessions. At the conclusion of each treatment session there are also home assignments for the parent to complete with their child. This should be instilled in the therapy regimen from the initial contact. However, in the end, parents will decide whether or not they will become part of the child's therapy; we sometimes hear, "Isn't that what I'm paying you to do?"

Children in Denial

Older children sometimes are in denial and don't want to be in therapy. They need therapy, but confronting their stuttering can seem to be just too much for them to handle. These young clients want their stuttering to go away but don't want to deal with it directly. This is not a good prognostic indicator. Often, a five- or six-session period of trial therapy may be proposed as an intermediate step to give therapy a try. But, unfortunately, their stuttering often has to worsen before the client sees the need and agrees to come to therapy. It is not uncommon for teens to deny their stuttering even throughout high school. But as they mature and begin to think about preparing for college or for a career, they come to realize that they need help. Waiting for the child to be ready for therapy is not always comfortable for anyone. Sometimes, years of suffering ensue before the client is ready. The longer the stuttering persists, the harder it is to overcome, not impossible, but just a bigger challenge as the habit strength and social repercussions of stuttering become more firmly established. There rarely are quick fixes to stuttering in speech therapy, but being "ready" is a critical component for a successful outcome.

For some children who are aware of their stuttering, denial is a strategy to avoid dealing with it. They deny that they stutter or deny that it bothers them. The fear of confronting their stuttering is greater than the pain of living with the ridicule of others. Denying stuttering, or that it is upsetting, is the easier path for the child to take; easier than dealing it directly or indirectly. But, in almost all instances, denial is living a lie.

Despite being able to "see through" the lie, it is difficult to decide whether to pursue therapy right away in spite of the child's reaction. Although beginning therapy is usually the right course of action, the decision may result in even greater resistance to the idea of confronting stuttering. The penalty of stuttering is greater than the hope for its resolution. Sadly, experience has shown that forcing a child into therapy is not usually a fruitful strategy.

Often clients feel that nothing can be done to overcome their stuttering. Others are afraid to try because they fear that therapy will not work, and then there would be no hope left for them. Ironically, by keeping therapy as an option, but not enrolling right away, it remains a viable option in their mind. Whereas trying it and failing would dash all hope.

Defining Success

For many for whom stuttering has become deeply engrained, no degree of disfluency is tolerable or acceptable. To be a "normal" speaker, the client often feels that he must have perfect fluency. This perspective is understandable as much of his experience in life has been having his speech disfluencies pointed out to him as being a personal shortcoming or flaw. In an attempt to compensate for this flaw, the client then feels he must be fluent all of the time; which of course is an unattainable goal. Building a tolerance for disfluency, stuttered, or normal disfluencies, is very beneficial. To not accept any disfluencies serves to heighten anxiety, which in turn increases muscular tension, which increases the likelihood of disfluency; a self-fulfilling prophecy.

So what should be the outcome of therapy? What end product are we to produce? Most consumers are looking to be able to speak without stuttering any more. For most older children, that is an unlikely outcome. Even as adults, we see that disfluencies continue, but become less frequent with time. As a consequence, we have a bit of selling to do; not selling in the sense of being deceptive, but selling in terms of developing an honest and realistic outcome that is communicated to and "bought" by the client and his parents. The outcome is a subject to be broached early on, like during the evaluation. This is sometimes a tough sell. Many parents have finally summoned the courage to confront their child's stuttering and now unhappily learn that the outcome of therapy might not be the end of their stuttering, but learning how to adjust to and manage it.

The Clinical Teaching Paradigm

How do clients learn in therapy? What is the role of the clinician? What are the responsibilities of the client and his parents in the therapeutic process?

A basic premise of stuttering therapy is for the client to learn to speak in different ways that better emulate the components of fluent speech production and ways that enable him to minimize his existing stuttering. Older children (beginning and intermediate levels of stuttering) are taught speaking techniques or *targets* that are to be practiced in progressively more challenging speaking situations and environments. Target use is complicated by the fear of stuttering and speaking anxieties, which are an integral part of this level of stuttering. Utilizing newly learned behaviors is exceedingly difficult under conditions when anxiety is present. The common human response is to revert back to old behaviors when anxiety strikes. This phenomenon appears to happen without the client's conscious recognition. When the client is asked why he did not use the new target, the response is frequently, *"I guess I forgot."* He intended to use the new target, but under the stress of anxiety he reverted back to his old speech habit.

Speech targets usually address the components of stuttering that are dysfunctional. For example, if the client's vocal folds are tightly adducted and no air is able to be exhaled for speech, a target will be prescribed that serves to overcome that issue. The client learns to replace the dysfunctional speaking behavior with the new target. Although a fairly simple and straightforward undertaking, the task is usually significantly complicated by the client's apprehension and fears.

The learning paradigm can be enhanced by two relatively simply strategies: preparation and reflection. Preparation involves directing the client's attention to what he is expected to learn. The 60 seconds it takes to describe what the client is going to learn before starting an activity usually pay big dividends. Anyone's awareness (and therefore his learning) is heightened by being told what to expect and what to look for. This anticipation increases the client's awareness of what he experiences. In doing so, the client's perceptions are guided or directed to specific aspects of the experience. For example, the clinician might explain to the client, *"We're going to make some phone calls and I'd like you to pay special attention to your speech just as you begin to speak right after the person says 'hello.' I think you see that you take a quick and deep inhalation of air that starts you off in an incorrect way. Let's make the first call and see if you notice what I'm talking about."*

Usually, clients are not aware of all of their speaking behaviors in stressful situations. But by drawing attention to this specific behavior, the client becomes aware of his maladaptive reaction in the speaking situation. Awareness is the first step in changing it. It is unlikely that this would have been noticed without anticipating it. Everyone can find a way to ignore information that "isn't flattering"; this is the ego's way of protecting us; shielding us for things that are painful.

As a result, being made aware of those behaviors is sometimes confrontational and uncomfortable and many clients will go to great lengths not to have to deal with it. However, guided confrontation is the means of overcoming those difficult aspects, and awareness is the first step. It usually makes it more palatable to the client if comments are made as objectively as possible. Talk about the behaviors, not the person. You might say, *"I noticed the speech rate increased right after she answered the call,"* instead of *"You started speaking too fast right after she answered the phone."* Clients are sometimes more open to clinician comments when they do not feel threatened or blamed. Discussing behaviors in objective (nonpersonal) terms is one means of promoting that. However, later on, after the client is better able to discuss his behaviors more openly, using *"you* language" becomes an important part of designating responsibility to the client for his actions and behaviors. Gauge the client's receptiveness to *"you* language" by his willingness to discuss his behaviors. Remember also that there's an important distinction to be made between responsibility and blame for behaviors. Clients do not feel that it is fair to be *blamed* for things they feel are out of their control, but they are *responsible* for managing them effectively.

The clinician's role in the clinical teaching paradigm is to be the guide or coach. Many clinicians have expressed concern that clients know more about their stuttering than the clinician does. This is true. They've spent much more time with it than the clinician and they know much more about it. However, what they believe is not always accurate, and there is much every client has yet to learn about his stuttering. Even the best professional athletes have coaches. The best tennis players, for example, all have coaches. When it comes to playing a game of tennis, the athlete can beat his coach hands down. So why does a player need a coach that is not as good a player as he is? What the coach (and in stuttering therapy, the clinician) brings is the ability to see the player from a perspective that the player himself cannot. The coach knows the game and how to play, but can provide feedback to the player that he is unable to see from his perspective on the court. Analogously, the clinician knows about stuttering, but can offer feedback from a perspective that is not available to the client.

Giving Feedback

Many clinicians underestimate the importance of giving meaningful feedback during and after therapy activities. Although saying, "*Good job*!" provides the client with a general, positive reassurance relative to his performance, it falls woefully short of the potential for communicating the information necessary to be meaningful or making clinical teaching/learning effective. What specifically about the client's response was good? What do we want the client to learn from the activity and his performance? Clinicians can maximize their clinical teaching ability by incorporating three feedback components into their teaching strategy—giving instructions, maintaining a single focus, and summarizing the client's performance.

1. Instructions. Instructions set the stage for what is expected of the client. Instructions should be relatively brief, yet explain the intent and purpose of the activity, while describing what the client is to do. Instructions should take only 20 to 30 seconds to complete. Spending time covering every nuance and possible outcome is likely not working as efficiently as you can and may only confuse the client. Be succinct and respect therapy time as the client's time to practice and learn. If the client misunderstands the instructions, it usually is fairly simple to redirect him.

Begin by explaining the purpose of the activity in terms of your expectations of the client's performance, challenges he will likely face, and how the activity fits into the overall treatment plan. When a client understands the rationale and significance of what he is being asked to do, his motivation and learning will both be enhanced. If the activity entails using a speech target, model the target while instructing the client. This shows the client what is expected of him in addition having it explained to him verbally. The power of modeling is hard to overestimate. Succinctly explain how the patient is to use any materials provided for the activity. Consider having the client demonstrate his understanding of what is expected on the first item of the activity before actually beginning. This enables the clinician to assess his comprehension of the task and provide further instruction as necessary. Last, inform the client of the parameter of the task that he will be evaluated on.

For example, the clinician might say, "*Next we're going to read some sentences and I'd like you to use your "stretches" on the first sound of the first word of each sentence. I've notice that the beginning of words is the biggest trouble spot, so that's why I'd like to focus on that. Listen as I show you what to do. 'I------------I want some ice cream.' Did you hear my stretch at the very beginning? You say the same thing I did, and then we'll start reading the sentences.*"

2. Focus on One Thing. Over the years, my daughter has had several coaches while playing baseball throughout her childhood. A few of her coaches stood out as being markedly better than the others. At batting practice, some coaches would give the instruction to, "*Keep your eyes on the ball.*" After the pitch and subsequent swing, the coach provided corrective feedback on a raft of things *other than* watching the ball! "*Keep your elbow up.*" "*Bend your knees more.*" "*Move your weight from your back to your front foot as you swing.*" Although all of this feedback was indeed valid, none of it dealt with what he had instructed her to do: keeping her eyes on the ball! As a consequence, she had no idea how she had done at what the coach specifically asked her to do. As a result, children (and adults) begin to feel that they are not good at batting (or using speech targets); they learned from their coach that just about everything that they are doing is wrong and end up feel defeated and discouraged.

The good coaches stayed focused on task. When instructed to, "*Keep your eyes on the ball,*" all of the coach's feedback was directed to that specific task. Were there other things that needed to be fixed? Certainly! But staying focused on one thing at a time is the best strategy to promote success. The batter could go home feeling like he had done *something* right—"*I kept my eye on the ball and the coach said I did a really good job*!"

Whether working with children or adults, focusing on a single target is usually preferable, even with long-standing clients. Try not to allow yourself to be distracted by other behaviors that also require some work. Therapy is a process. Take note of the other things that need to be worked on and incorporate them in therapy at a later time when they can receive the full focus of an activity.

3. Summary. At the conclusion of an activity, summarize the client's performance by commenting on his successes, things that he did very well, and challenges that still lie ahead. The summary enables the clinician to tell the client what he should have learned from the activity, further guiding his learning. Putting his current performance into the perspective of his improvements to date and what challenges still lie ahead, the clinician can motivate the client and help him understand the process of his therapy. Giving a summary also is a means of smoothly transitioning to the next activity, a marker that the activity is now complete and we are moving to the next one.

The clinician might say, "*You used your stretches perfectly on 8 of the 10 sentences you read. I'm so impressed. I let you know when the stretches weren't quite long enough and you quickly made them better. Sometimes when we hurry something it doesn't work as well and I want to be sure that these stretches work for you. I think we should try using stretches while we talk about your soccer game. You are really working hard to put your stretches to work for you. Let's put them to work in the next activity."*

Sharing the Plan and Demonstrating Success

Children and their parents can get more from therapy when they understand what they are doing, why they are doing it, the direction therapy is leading them, and where they currently are in the overall schema. Discussing the overall design and course of therapy helps clients to understand and become involved in the treatment plan designed for them. A deeper understanding of therapy enables them to be better observers and better reporters of events which transpire outside the therapy room. Similarly, clients are more likely to be motivated when they better recognize the significance of small changes in their speech. Making the client and parents part of the plan subtly communicates the message that they are part of the process, rather than thinking it is the clinician's responsibility to fix the stuttering.

From the beginning, review the "master plan" of therapy with the client and his family, explaining the significance of each of the components of therapy. Show the client, based upon his performance level, where along the path he currently is in therapy. Clients are educated by the clinician sharing her observations, thoughts, and specific experiences with the client's stuttering.

The Overall Schema

The developmental level of the child's stuttering helps determine the therapeutic approach to be selected. As previously pointed out, caution must be taken not to draw the child's attention to his disfluencies in any way that could be thought of as negative. As a consequence, therapy approaches for children in the borderline and beginning levels of stuttering require the clinician's discretion in working on the child's speech. For children aware of their stuttering, a more direct approach typically is chosen. In either case, the outcome goal of therapy is natural fluency.

The underlying premise of therapy is predicated on two thoughts. One notion is that the child's fluency can be facilitated indirectly by manipulating elements of his speaking environment and remediating any developmental delays that might interfere with the function of the speech system. The second premise is the belief that children can make their speech more fluent (smoother) when reinforced to do so. Without specific instruction, young children who stutter can often improve their speech fluency in an attempt to please others, especially their parents or speech pathologist.

For children having progressed into intermediate or advanced levels of stuttering, treating the stuttering more directly provides tools for the client to manage stuttering moments more adeptly and learn to speak in ways which better emulate normal speech production. The clients are taught techniques (or targets) that shorten the duration disfluencies and lessen muscular effort that has become part of the stuttering pattern.

These targets serve as tools to empower the client to speak more fluently. Many of the child's stuttered speaking habits are replaced with targets based on normal, fluent speech production.

> **Clinical Insight:** Sometimes, when a new technique or target is introduced in therapy, it appears to be very effective at first and the child's fluency is dramatically improved. Everyone is elated. However, after a short time, old habits can infiltrate the new technique and it inevitably takes its place among the other "new techniques" previously introduced in therapy. This is frustrating for all involved. Avoid therapy becoming a "new target of the week" proposition. Spending the time necessary to build a strong foundation for each target will help ensure that they remain effective for a much longer time. Keep therapy focused; periodically review targets to be sure the client continues to use them correctly and that they are still fresh in his mind.

Treatment Activities

Like therapy for any communication disorder, therapeutic activities in stuttering therapy with children play a central role in clinical teaching and learning. Activities provide the clinical environment intended to enable the client to develop specific skills while various elements or parameters are manipulated to adjust to level of difficulty of the task. Task difficulty is often determined by the success rate attained by the client engaged in the activity. There usually are several parameters to each activity that serve as tools by which the clinician can modify and adjust the level of an activity to appropriately challenge the client. The challenge must be sufficient for the client to maintain a reasonable level of success. In other words, an activity should be neither too difficult nor too easy to facilitate the client's learning optimally. A success rate of 75 to 90% generally is considered the most favorable. If the client's performance level is lower, consider changing one parameter to make the activity less difficult. If the client is getting more the 90% correct, it usually is prudent to make the activity harder. Activities are also utilized to help clients discover things about their speaking skills or challenge the beliefs they hold and their feelings about their stuttering.

The clinician has the responsibility to move their client through therapy as quickly as possible. Spending too much time on tasks on which the client is already successful may not be the most effective use of therapy time. However, most clients benefit from activities designed to keep existing skills sharp; this promotes carryover and confidence. Therefore, it may be prudent to assign "mastered" activities as homework or use them as warm-ups at the beginning of each treatment session.

Activity Parameters

The level of challenge of most stuttering therapy activities can be manipulated by varying factors such as the physical speaking environment, the complexity of the utterance, and the client's perception of the degree of difficulty it represents (see Chapter 1 for a discussion of these parameters). It is important that activities enable clients to be cognizant of their success, but also be aware that there is still room for improvement. This can be accomplished by systematically varying the following parameters of an activity in a systematic way.

Environmental Variables

The effect of the speaking environment differs widely among people who stutter. Generally, clients who stutter experience more difficulty talking on the phone, giving presentations, speaking to authority figures, speaking under time pressure, being interrupted, asking questions in class, and saying their name introducing themselves to strangers. Most who stutter see their stuttering to be greatly diminished when they are speaking when alone, speaking in unison with someone else, while reading aloud, talking to a pet, or when whispering. Again, individual circumstances vary, so it is important to work with the parents to determine the critical variables in any specific child's environment.

For many children who stutter, stuttering frequency is often increased by noise and auditory distractions in their immediate speaking environment. Each client's tolerance for noise should be evaluated individually, as specific sounds can be more or less distracting for some than others. Noise disruptions can be simulated in therapy using recorded background sounds, such as cafeteria noise. Other auditory distractions can be momentary and unpredictable, as opposed to the relative consistency of cafeteria noise. Noises can distract the client's ability to monitor his speech production, interfere with the thought processes, or cause them to stress their speech system in trying to compensate for the disruption by talking louder or faster. It is interesting that when clients cannot hear their own speech production (such as while listening to white noise) their fluency improves. However, in general, auditory competition such as speaking in a noisy environment, stresses speakers. To compensate, the child who stutters should focus more attention on the motor facets of speaking, rather than attempt to overpower noise by speaking louder.

Being interrupted while speaking is relatively commonplace in our culture and can sometimes be annoying. Interrupting the child can be used as another environmental variable that can be manipulated to challenge the child's developing fluency skills. The clinician intentionally asks questions or interjects ideas as the child is speaking. Relatedly, hurrying the client to speak more quickly is another form of environmental stress which disrupts the client's attempts to communicate. Using gestures, body language and prompts to "hurry along" enable the clinician to add stress to the child's speaking environment. All children commonly experience speaking situations in which they perceive the need to speak more quickly. Children who stutter need to be able to deal with pressured situations like this to be successful outside the treatment room.

Children also often vie for the attention of adult listeners at home and at school. Competition to be heard usually results in speaking louder and often more quickly to their intended audience. Incorporating another child or sibling into therapy activities may enable the clinician to simulate increased competition for speaking time in the clinic room.

Note that parents initially are advised to manipulate these variables in just the opposite direction, attempting to create an environment that is optimal to facilitate fluency in the home. Over time, parents may be asked to manipulate these variables at home to mimic the treatment conditions in the therapy room.

> **Clinical Insight:** It is not uncommon for children who stutter to become quite fluent in the therapy room with their clinician. Some clients demonstrate near 100% fluency and it is tempting to discharge the child from therapy. Before discharging the client, however, discuss the child's fluency in his other speaking environments to determine if his fluency in therapy is a consequence of not sufficiently challenging the child, or if the client is truly nearing the time to be discharged. The performance in the treatment room often exceeds the client's performance in other situations because the clinician may have created a speaking environment that is "too optimal" and differs too much from the child's real world.

Asking questions, or even changing the way questions are asked, of the child who stutters can represent another variable. Asking for specific information often leaves fewer options for a response. For example asking, "*What's your name*?" or "*What did you have for lunch today*?" do not afford the same latitude in answering as does the question, "*What would you like to do on Saturday*?" or "*Do you think the Panthers will win their first hockey game?*" Asking questions in a way that permits flexibility in how the child responds reduces stress for clients who stutter. For some, this represents a significant and critical difference.

Sample Treatment Plans

Younger Children

With children who stutter it is important that a parent or caregiver observe and be an active part of treatment sessions. In settings such as the schools, this is a difficult obstacle to overcome. Another approach might be to incorporate frequent communications as a part of therapy, providing narrative explanations, homework and periodic phone contacts or face-to-face meetings with parents. Therapy only within the context of the isolation of the therapy room is a more difficult path because there is no one to guide the child in carrying over the work in the therapy room to other environments.

Also, therapy benefits when information about the child's speech performance outside therapy is available. With training, parents can provide a broader picture of the challenges faced by the child in everyday life. Reports of the settings, types of disfluency, frequency, and details such as the number of iterations of repetitions are helpful in understanding the true scope of the child's difficulty. Given these parameters to measure, parents of children who stutter begin looking at their child's speech difficulty in more objective, and less emotional ways. As a consequence, their natural reactions to disfluencies become less emotionally charged, which the child may perceive as meaning his stuttering is less distressing for to his parents.

Children often are privy to parental discussions about their speech. It therefore is important that words be chosen that do not denote exasperation or anything negative relating to how the child speaks. This can take some thought and practice.

Structuring Session Activities

Younger children usually require more activities of shorter duration to maintain their attention and active participation. Five to 10 minutes for each activity may be a reasonable starting point. Sessions usually begin by reviewing an important feature of the therapeutic regimen. In Table 2–3, the session begins with the client demonstrating his proficiency using smooth speech. A secondary purpose of the activity is to refresh and guide the client's production of the desired response—smooth speech.

The second activity uses the same target into a more challenging environment by manipulating the speaking mode; changing from telling a story to expressing opinions.

Table 2–3. Sample Lesson Plan for Younger Children

Activity	Goal	Behavioral Objective
1. Warm-Up: Using smooth speech during a dialogue	Target use in telling a story	Telling a story from a wordless picture book for 3 minutes, the client will maintain smooth speech with 85% accuracy.
2. Using smooth speech in conversation	Target use in conversation	While discussing the benefits of dogs as pets, the client will use smooth speech with 75% accuracy, with clinician cueing.
3. Identifying speech bumps	Identify and objectively describe disfluencies	While monitoring the clinician telling a story, the client will identify the clinician's speech bumps with 90% accuracy.
4. Using smooth speech under time pressure	Target use when pressured to speak more quickly	Given a set of picture cards, the client will utter a sentence about the action portrayed in as many pictures as possible within 10 seconds, using smooth speech with 70% accuracy.
Homework: Using smooth speech at home	Speech target use in reading	During dinner each evening, the client will read his homework assignments for the day using smooth speech.

The task uses more resources in that the client must formulate his own opinions instead of verbalizing a prescribed story as in the warm-up activity.

In the third activity, the clinician shifts gears and asks the "student" to become the "teacher" as a means of working toward developing his self-monitoring skills using the smooth speech target. The client listens to the clinician's speech and identifies bumps that the clinician intentionally interjects into her speech.

The final activity uses time pressure to raise the level of challenge of the activity. The child is shown pictures and must describe the main action being depicted within the time constraints of the activity. A stopwatch may provide additional visual feedback for the client.

Finally, to set the expectation that smooth speech is not just to be used in the therapy room, a daily assignment is provided in a context that requires minimal extra work on behalf of the family. Asking the parents to make notes about the child's performance each day supplies helpful feedback to the clinician.

Older Children

Generally speaking, stuttering in older children may have continued to develop; therefore therapy is structured to work more directly on stuttering behaviors. At this level of stuttering development, children need tools to be able to manage stuttering moments and deal more directly with disfluencies. In the design of therapy, the aforementioned elements of complexity, environmental variables, response rate, and utility apply to older children as well (see Table 2–3).

In general, older children can attend longer to activities and stay focused on their target use. Therapy consists more on using targets in a variety of speaking modalities. Sessions usually begin with a warm-up activity, like piano lessons often begin with the pupil playing scales. The intent is to re-orient the client to therapy as a transition from the activity in which he was previously involved. The second purpose is to ensure that he can properly use the targets. Because many clients don't practice outside of therapy, in this way the clinician determines the client's current level of proficiency.

In the sample lesson plan (Table 2–4), the client begins by describing a picture using slow rate or Turtle Talk. It is important that the clinician model the rate the child is expected to use. Modeling is a very effective clinical tool. Frequent feedback helps the child know that he is using the desired rate. Feedback should be both corrective when the client is not performing as required, and complimentary to reinforce his correct production.

The second activity carries the same target (slow rate) into a more challenging mode; conversation. Pictures that are exciting to the child, perhaps action sports or humorous incidents may challenge the client's target use even further.

The third activity practices a different target, Easy Starts, in reading. Children who have difficulty initiating utterances because of their stuttering need a reliable means to be able to start speaking. The speaking mode, reading aloud, makes the task less challenging than other modes, enabling the client to focus more on producing targets effectively.

Next, the challenge for using Easy Starts is increased by inviting a new person into the session to ask the client questions, to which he responds using his targets. The clini-

Table 2–4. Sample Lesson Plan for Older Children

Activity	Goal	Behavioral Objective
1. Warm-Up: Using slow rate while describing a picture	Target use describing a picture	Presented with a series of pictures the client will describe each picture using slow rate with 85% accuracy.
2. Using slow rate in a conversation	Target use in conversation	While discussing things to take on a picnic at the beach, the client will use slow rate with 75% accuracy.
3. Using Easy Starts in reading	Target use in reading	While reading individual sentences, the client will use Easy Starts on the first sound of the first word of each sentence with 90% accuracy.
4. Using Easy Starts to answer questions	Target use speaking with an unfamiliar partner	Answering questions from a novel communication partner, the client will use Easy Starts with 70% accuracy.
Homework: Using Easy Starts at school	Target use in the classroom	The client will ask one question in class each day using Easy Starts.

cian may develop some subtle signs or gestures to cue the client toward better target use, should his performance level falter.

Homework is assigned to carry target use into the child's environment. It is often useful to negotiate the specifics of homework, in terms of the where and when, with the client. This makes him part of the decision-making process and helps prevent assigning work that the child is not willing to do.

Clinical Insight: Sometimes when using games as activities in therapy, the game becomes more important than the therapeutic goal of the activity. Games can motivate children to participate in speech work activities, but not always for the desired reasons. Much of speech therapy requires mental processing to learn. Just getting the desired response from the client is not always enough. It is preferable for the client to be aware of what he is doing and reflect upon his performance to optimize its learning effectiveness. Therapy activities are not always inherently interesting for clients, but when a game activity becomes the primary focus, it can diminish learning potential and thereby the effectiveness of therapy. It's not just the "doing" that matters, it's being aware of what you're doing that really counts.

Support Resources

The Internet

The amount of information on stuttering currently available on the Internet has been a mixed blessing. It has enabled far better access to information for many. Unfortunately, not all the information is factual or from reputable sources. It is sometimes difficult for parents to evaluate the credibility of Internet sources.

For many who stutter, the Internet has given them a voice, a vehicle to express their thoughts about their stuttering with others. It is far less daunting to express themselves electronically, via E-mail, blogs, chat rooms, or on Web sites and there is not the risk of stuttering in the process. These electronic means of expression have enabled people who stutter to communication more openly and more freely. Clinicians should consider using E-mail as a vehicle to encourage children to discuss their speech and as a means of reporting on their homework assignments. It also may be an important line of communication with parents unable to attend treatment session.

Everyone who stutters has opinions about it. Stuttering has an unfortunate history of misinformation and folklore, and some postings on the Internet serve to fuel these misunderstandings and inaccuracies. Additionally, the Internet marketplace includes many remedies, cures, and other boondoggles relating to overcoming stuttering. It can be difficult for the naïve reader or vulnerable client to distinguish between reliable and questionable information sources. Credible Internet resources such as the Stuttering Foundation of America (http://www.stutteringhelp.org) can be important building blocks in helping families learn about stuttering problems.

Organizations/Support Groups

Parents experience a range of emotions relating to their child's disfluencies. As a consequence, it often is helpful to have positive, credible support resources to help them address their fears and anxieties about stuttering. Speech pathologists should recognize that, in our role as a service provider, we can be perceived as having a financial interest in promoting our services, the potential for a conflict of interest. Additionally, the client is not our child, and a parent's angst and determination to do what is best comes with different emotions, greater intensity, and zeal. But a characteristic of childhood stuttering is its uncertainty and unpredictability; questions about childhood stuttering abound, even among the experts in stuttering therapy.

Parents are concerned about their child's future if he continues to stutter. These are rational fears, and although speech pathologists can offer parents reassurance, we can neither predict the future nor guarantee that the child will not be ridiculed about their speech. A parent's role is to protect their child and the threat of stuttering is rarely taken lightly. Credible information is one element that can help parents defend their child against stuttering. However, there is not an abundance of factual information yet available; at least not enough to quell their fears. Similar credible support sources come from groups such as the National Stuttering Association (http://www.westutter.org) and Friends (http://www.friendswhostutter.org).

"Googling" is frequently used to access information. However, there are too few filters available through which information passes to determine the relevance or credibility of the information available. There are some astonishing materials on the Internet about stuttering, some of which are truly regrettable. Organizations, such as those mentioned above, have worked diligently to make current, reputable, and objective information available for everyone, particularly people who stutter and parents of children who stutter.

Many people become easy prey to miracle cures and quick fixes out frustration with what they have experienced, their hope regarding what might be, and fears that there may be nothing available to help them. These vulnerabilities soften them to believe information they want to hear.

References

DeNil, L. F., Kroll, R. M., Lafaille, S. J., & Houle, S. (2003). A positron emission tomography study of short- and long-term treatment effects on functional brain activation in adults who stutter. *Journal of Fluency Disorders*, *28*, 357–380.

Guitar, B. (2006). *Stuttering: An integrated approach to its nature and treatment* (p. 167). Baltimore, MD: Lippincott Williams & Wilkins.

Starkweather, C. W. (1987). *Fluency and stuttering*. Englewood Cliffs, NJ: Prentice-Hall.

Yairi, E., & Ambrose, N. G. (2005). *Early childhood stuttering*. Austin, TX: Pro-Ed.

CHAPTER

3

Stuttering in Adolescents and Adults

Working with stuttering in its more advanced form changes the expected outcome, and consequently our perspectives on treatment. When working with children who stutter, there is the hope of regaining natural fluency. With adolescents and adults, the objective of therapy is learning to manage stuttering in ways that will enable the client to participate fully in all work, school, family, and social activities while speaking confidently without embarrassment.

The client's feelings, emotions, and beliefs about their stuttering complicate treatment significantly. Therapy addresses both the client's speech and the emotional components of his stuttering. The treatment program reflects this as it becomes a combination of speech therapy and counseling.

Stuttering therapy with adults is as much an art as a science. Although the science of therapy is based in our treatment philosophy, speech techniques, and counseling goals, the art of therapy comes in applying them to the specific needs of the individual client.

Chapter Outline

- An Overview of Adolescent and Adult Stuttering
- Assessing Adolescents and Adults Who Stutter
- Speech Characteristics of Adolescents and Adults Who Stutter
- Affective Characteristics of Stuttering
- Treatment Approaches
- Working with Emotions: Anxiety, Fear, Negative Past Experiences
- Working with Covert Stuttering
- Determining a Starting Point for Therapy
- Therapy Techniques (Targets)
  - Fluency-Enhancing Targets
  - Stuttering-Modification Targets
- Signs of Progress in Therapy
- The Structure of Individual Therapy Sessions
- Task Modes in Therapy
- Sample Therapy Session
- Organizations and Support Groups

An Overview of Adolescent and Adult Stuttering

When planning a trip or vacation it's important to consider the things you would like to do and see and then establish a schedule or itinerary for the journey to ensure you accomplish all that you set out to do. If you are driving, you might find a map (or GPS) and directions are helpful to get you to your destination. The intent of this chapter on the overview of therapy for adults who stutter is to provide clinicians with a broad map and general directions for therapy. Unlike a vacation in which there usually are a specific number of days you will be spending away from home, the therapy itinerary is governed less by a specific number of treatment sessions, but more by the needs of the client and speed at which he makes progress. This is to say that clients advance at their own pace. However, it is the responsibility of the clinician to move the client as rapidly as possible.

There are three overarching goals of stuttering therapy for adolescents and adults. They include:

- learning to better manage and minimize existing instances of stuttering,
- acquiring speaking behaviors that will enhance natural speech fluency, and
- learning to cope with the feelings, attitudes, emotions, and beliefs that have developed in response to stuttering.

These three objectives are addressed concurrently throughout therapy. Experience finds that some areas are more difficult to treat than others, usually the feelings and emotional reactions to stuttering. Consequently, a meaningful starting point in therapy may be to offer the client a means of gaining some control over his stuttering. Learning that stuttering can be manipulated is an empowering feeling, as clients who struggle with their speech feel victimized by their stuttering, as though there is nothing that can be done when stuttering "strikes" them, taking control of their efforts to speak. These three components constitute the core of the treatment program, but vary in relative proportion as therapy progresses. Figure 3–1 illustrates how the proportion of time devoted to each component is adjusted over the course of therapy. In the beginning, more time is spent on stuttering management issues, with some effort dedicated to fluency enhancement, and relatively little work on emotional issues. Toward the conclusion of therapy the proportion shifts with relatively little time being spent working on stuttering management or fluency enhancement, as the focus of therapy now emphasizes the affective aspects of stuttering. Learning to control stuttering is empowering, motivating, and makes a notable difference in the problem. This makes it a good place to begin therapy. Developing enough trust in the clinician to be able to discuss personal feelings and difficult emotions takes time; consequently it should be expected that being able to work effectively in this affective area would come later in the therapeutic process after trust and mutual understanding have been built.

Most adolescents and adults who stutter do not yet recognize that many of their speaking behaviors invite increased frequency of stuttering and disfluency. The behaviors most commonly related to anxieties include speaking at a rapid rate, abrupt voice

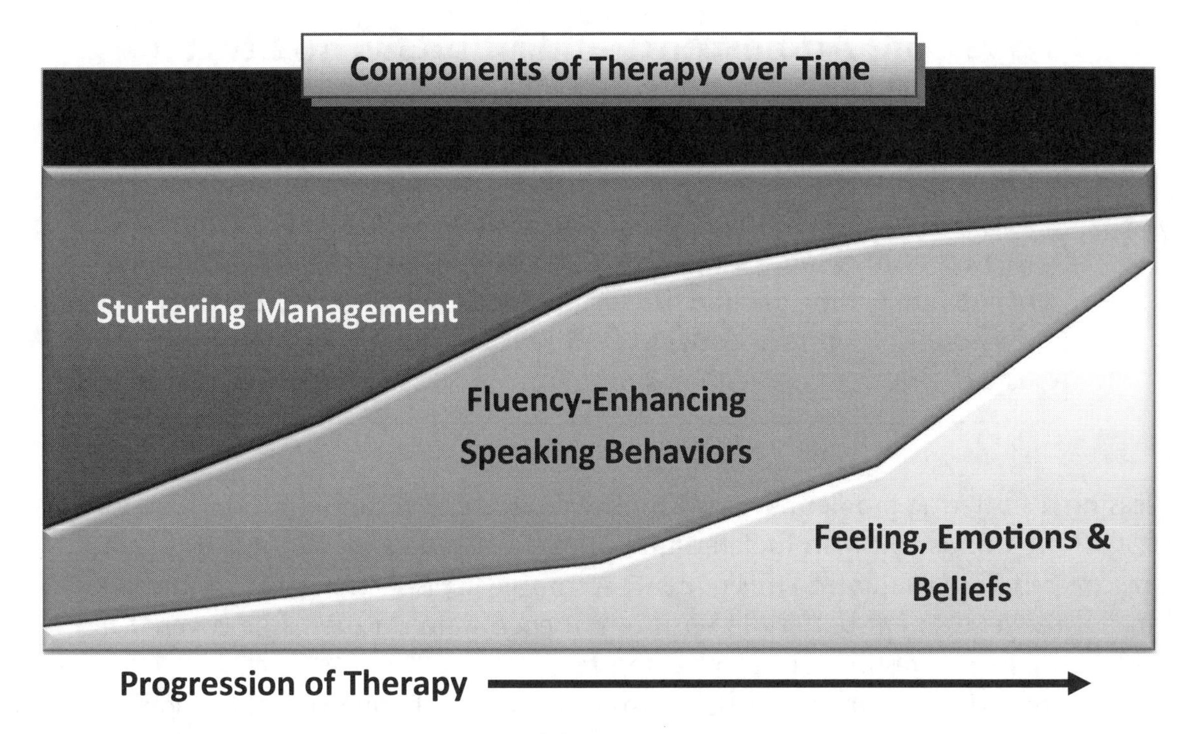

Figure 3–1. Relative proportions of therapy components as treatment progresses.

onsets, and excessive muscular effort and struggle articulating sounds. The client often has only limited awareness of these behaviors and is not cognizant of how they create even more stuttering. Ironically, the client's attempts to overpower his stuttering usually result in increased levels of disfluency. Learning "fluency-compatible" speaking patterns frees the client from a good deal of stuttering and enhances his natural fluency. Speech is an ongoing, forward moving, almost effortless sequence of motor behaviors. Fluency-compatible speaking behaviors work to correctly apportion the appropriate amount of effort necessary to attain naturally fluent speech. With less muscular effort and using a slow rate, coordination and movement sequences are naturally enhanced.

Embarrassing experiences unfortunately are very effective in creating fears and anxiety about speaking and stuttering. It is the fear and anxiety about being embarrassed that result in more stuttering. These emotions trigger thoughts and bodily responses that increase muscular tension; this makes stuttering more likely. Over time, these experiences and emotions become internalized into the thought processes of those who stutter. Stuttering in this advanced stage is significantly more difficult to treat. Treatment therefore must address both the speech characteristics and the affective characteristics of stuttering as they are intricately interwoven into the fabric of the disorder.

The intent of this section is to provide an overview of the treatment process. More detailed information about each of the three components of stuttering therapy follows later in this chapter in the section on Treatment Approaches. But therapy starts with an inventory of the characteristics of the client's stuttering.

Assessing Adolescents and Adults Who Stutter

> **Clinical Insight:** Assessment is a process that continues over the duration of the therapeutic relationship. Like a good friend, there is always something more to be learned about the client. It usually takes time to build the trust needed to move a relationship (personal or clinical) forward and reveal more of the personal aspects which underlie their stuttering.

Assessing a stuttering problem begins with the desired end result in mind. First, develop a list of all the things you wish to determine from the assessment. What is it that needs to be discovered from evaluating this patient? A sample list is seen below in Table 3–1. Then plan out the assessment battery to ensure that each item on the list is covered through observation, formal testing, or in conversation.

It is important to establish the diagnosis of stuttering if you are seeking some form of third-party reimbursement. Many third parties also require a rating of the severity of the stuttering and a prognosis for improvement. In other instances, the likely cause of stuttering is an important criterion, whether the stuttering is "developmental" or related to a neurologic incident.

> **Clinical Insight:** People generally seek help because they are unable to resolve the problem themselves. Sometimes they are lost, sometimes confused. Many people who stutter have tried on their own and not succeeded whereas others are looking to be guided or mentored; some looking to be "fixed." Understanding the client's perspective better enables us to meet his needs.

It is also important to learn how the patient perceives his stuttering and what he wishes to gain from therapy. People seek our services because they are unable to resolve their stuttering problems on their own. To satisfy our consumer (the patient), we need to understand what he wants, even if what he?? are looking for is unrealistic. Interviewing the client gives us that information and much more.

It is important to know if there is a family history of stuttering and whether the stuttering of these relatives persisted or resolved. Research to date indicates that this is perhaps the best indicator of the outcome for the present client's stuttering. However, by early adulthood, the likelihood of stuttering persisting is extremely high. But knowing there are other relatives who stutter can provide insight into how the family perceives and reacts to stuttering.

Table 3–1. Interview Topics

Information to be Determined	Questions	Significance
Background of Stuttering	When did it begin? Does anyone else in your family stutter? Do they still stutter? How has your stuttering changed over time? Have you had therapy before? What did you learn? How effective was it?	This information helps determine if stuttering developed in a usual fashion and how it progressed over time. Prior therapy may provide a starting point for treatment now and determine the client's disposition toward speech therapy.
What the client is looking for	What brings you here today? How do you think your life would be different if you didn't stutter? What are your expectations for your speech at the conclusion of therapy?	Provides insight into the patient's perceptions of the problem(s). This helps the clinician to satisfy the patient's needs and can serve to shape realistic expectations of a treatment outcome. Therapy is presented in terms of how it addresses the patient's goals.
Impact/ Handicapping Effects	Do you talk about your stuttering to other people? How does stuttering hold you back at work and in your social relationships? How do you feel after when you stutter?	Helpful to assess the overall severity of the stuttering. The life decisions the client allows his stuttering to influence is a measure of the overall handicap of the stuttering, rather than only relying on the overt features of the stuttering behaviors
Outcomes	What do you hope the outcome of therapy will be?	It's important that therapy paint a realistic outcome for the client. Some client's are more realistic than others, but this question reveals where the client's thoughts are at this time.
Knowledge of Stuttering	Are there particular words or sounds that are more difficult for you to say? Are there specific situations in which you consistently have trouble? Do you find some people more difficult to talk to than others? What happens when you stutter? What do you think is the cause of your stuttering? What do you do when you don't want to stutter in a specific situation? Where does your stuttering take place, in your throat, mouth? Do you feel tension when you stutter? Where is it focused? Are there times when you don't stutter?	The client's knowledge of their stuttering can reveal their openness to talk about it. It also reveals whether they perceive their stuttering objectively or emotionally. Some of their feelings and beliefs about stuttering also may surface in this discussion.

continues

Table 3–1. *continued*

Information to be Determined	Questions	Significance
Speech Techniques	Have you ever had therapy before? What did you do? What did you learn from it? What do you do when you want to be fluent or not stutter? What was hardest for you about the therapy?	Benefiting from previous experiences in therapy can provide insights for this current attempt to improve stuttering.

Stuttering rarely begins in adulthood. Learning about the development of the disorder provides insight into previous therapy attempts, how the stuttering has changed over time, and what the client knows (and doesn't know) about his stuttering; especially what he feels caused it. Part of therapy is educating the client about stuttering; misinformation usually causes needless angst and complications. We will want the client to be able to educate others about stuttering, and therefore he will need the best information and a script to be able to do so intelligently.

Clinical Insight: When stuttering begins in adulthood it is most likely related to a neurologic insult, such as a car accident, head injury, stroke, or drug overdose. In rare instances, stuttering results from psychological trauma. In some instances when stuttering first appears in adulthood, clients claim that they did not stutter as a child. Often the reality is that they were indeed quite disfluent as a child, but their disfluencies never rose to a level of concern. Yet others think of stuttering as blocking and struggling to speak in their childhood experience, even though they evidenced disfluencies in their speech, their symptoms did not include blocks. They consequently conclude that they did not stutter previously.

Most clients are also aware of specific words, sounds, situations, and speaking environments that pose challenges for them. This information is important because these concerns may be specifically addressed in the treatment plan. The aim is to develop the client's confidence in his ability to articulate these sounds, thereby overcoming his fears.

The assessment further serves to document the characteristics of the client's stuttering at the time of the evaluation. This should include the type of disfluencies (blocks, repetitions, prolongations, etc.) the client displays, his secondary characteristics, and a description of his thoughts, feelings, and beliefs about his stuttering. Each of these categories is addressed in therapy and the assessment data can serve as a baseline. The clinician usually learns much more about the client's thoughts, feelings, and beliefs about stuttering through the course of therapy as he becomes more comfortable and trusting in the therapeutic relationship.

Experimenting with speech targets also provides valuable information. Initial targets are selected that address the predominant characteristics of the client's stuttering. For example, the airflow technique might be selected if laryngeal blocks are present; the pull-out technique might be tried with blockages that occur in the oral cavity. Testing the client's tolerance for speaking at a slow rate can also be telling. Many who stutter diminish the frequency and severity of their stuttering significantly just by speaking at a slower rate. However, in spite of the improved fluency, speaking slower seems almost repugnant to them. Many will maintain a slow rate only as long as requested. Others cannot maintain it for more than a few words before reverting back to their habitually quick speaking rate. Practically all clients express their dislike for speaking in this manner, despite its benefit to their fluency. The client's persistence and tolerance for speaking more slowly may be an indicator of the length of time they will be in therapy. Those who are disciplined enough to maintain a slow normal speaking rate and do not express the perception that it "does not feel normal" (or in some cases that it is worse than stuttering) have an advantage in the therapy to follow. A quick speaking rate usually is a reflection of underlying nervousness and anxiety. These emotions can distort the client's reality and perception of how different his speech sounds. For some, ironically, there is an element of comfort in their stuttering because, as much as the client doesn't like it, their stuttering is well known to them. Speaking in a manner in any way different than is their habit can easily be perceived as undesirable and clients are often unwilling to even try it. Therefore, successful techniques are those that reduce the frequency and severity of overt stuttering which the client will agree to use. Although other techniques may be introduced later in therapy, these targets may be good ones to begin with.

The clinician also needs to appreciate the client's expectations from therapy, what he is looking to accomplish. These expectations are often unrealistic, but serve as a place from which more realistic expectations can be molded. Part of educating the client may include learning to be more accepting of his stuttering and discovering that learning to manage fluency in any situation would be a satisfactory outcome.

Speech Characteristics of Adolescents and Adults Who Stutter

When inventorying behaviors, begin with the core features of stuttering. The core (overt) features of stuttering include repetitions, prolongations, blocks, and tremors. Repetitions are among the most common elements of stuttering; they may include repeated sounds, syllables, single-syllable words, and part-words. Repetitions of elements greater in length than a word usually are not considered to be stuttering, but are thought to be normal disfluencies. Repetitions are perhaps the most common behavior and are often thought to be how stuttering begins. A prolongation is the continuation of voicing or airflow that results when the cessation of movement of the articulators for a period of time during speech production. Prolongations usually last from a fraction to a few seconds in duration. Often, the whole body seems to freeze as the speaker prolongs the sound. Blocks are a total stoppage of voicing and airflow; they may occur at the level of the vocal folds or articulators. There is excessive muscular tension that restricts the movement of the vocal folds (laryngeal block), holding them in adducted position. As a result, the flow of exhaled air is blocked. Laryngeal blocks tense the vocal folds to the degree that very little or no air can escape, or sometimes air sporadically escapes in uncontrolled bursts. Blocks also can occur at the articulators (lingual or labial blocks). Lingual and labial blocks "freeze" the articulators; sound is sometimes present, but the client appears "stuck" and has difficulty moving his speech forward. Sometimes, there is so much muscular tension in the articulators that the jaw begins to quiver at a very rapid rate; this is referred to as a tremor.

Clients generally have a distinctive habit pattern of overt stuttering behaviors, but they may differ in the core features that comprise their stuttering. Much of stuttering therapy is directed at minimizing and eliminating the speech characteristics of stuttering. In advanced stages of stuttering, the overt characteristics are only a part of the problem. We will see that the client's feelings, emotions, and beliefs contribute to many of the overt stuttering symptoms.

Much of stuttering is not seen and, as such, often goes unaddressed. These covert characteristics of stuttering arguably are the more difficult side of the problem to work with because they are not visible. Yet, the covert features are a measure of the client's reactions to stuttering and his manner of coping with it. Not addressing them as part of therapy would be missing a key component of the problem and would likely contribute to eventual relapse of the problem.

Affective Characteristics of Stuttering

Adults and adolescents who stutter almost always have strong feelings about their speech. These feelings are understandable, natural reactions to the responses from others, which for most who stutter, become ingrained as a part of their personality and thought pattern.

At this advanced point of stuttering, feelings and emotions effect bodily changes and precipitate behaviors that serve to increase moments of stuttering. Basically, speaking anxieties work to increase muscle tension; for those who stutter, increased muscular tension is seen in the articulators and vocal folds. Speakers who stutter often try to force their way through their disfluencies, resulting in more struggle behaviors and leading to increased severity of the stuttering.

In response to their anxiety, most speakers increase speaking rate. For the person who stutters, increasing rate often serves to exceed the functional capacity of their speech mechanism, resulting in disfluency. Speech fluency breaks down in the same way that running down stairs increases the likelihood that you will trip and fall. Exceeding your body's functional capacity to descend a flight of stairs safely usually results in problems of timing, coordination, and accuracy of muscle movements. Analogously, speaking too fast can have the identical result for those who stutter. Most people who stutter significantly increase their fluency rather simply by speaking more slowly. But slowing speaking rate is more difficult than it seems. The body's natural reaction to anxiety by increasing rate happens reflexively or automatically. Maintaining a slow rate in this circumstance is a difficult challenge.

Clinical Perspective: For some who stutter you might think of disfluencies being related to trying to speak at a rate which is too fast for their oral motor system. Thinking about speech as a motor skill, there is often a speed (or range of speeds) that is optimal for movement. At that speed, movements proceed in a smooth, coordinated fashion with little to no interruption. Trying to move too quickly increases the risk of breakdown; moving too slowly distorts the result. Take riding a bike for example. When going too slowly, it can be difficult to keep your balance. Going too fast (like pedaling down a hill) increases the risk that even a small adjustment in steering will send you over the handlebars. If you consider a person who stutters as having an oral motor system that in some way is insufficient to keep up with the demands of the rapid movements of talking fast, you would expect that breakdowns would be more frequent during this condition. This would explain why slowing speaking rate improves fluency for most who stutter. It enables oral movements to be made at a speed that the oral mechanism is better able function.

Other responses to anxiety can include abrupt initiation of speaking, sudden gasps for air preceding feared words, forceful articulation of feared sounds, changing words, frequent use of interjections, poor eye contact when speaking, and several others. Sometimes, muscular tension appears in other parts of the body, such as fidgeting, knee jiggling, hyper-reflexivity and the like. It is these emotional components of stuttering that trigger instances of disfluency and other physical behaviors.

Treatment Approaches

Therapy for stuttering includes modifying and managing existing stuttering behaviors, learning new fluency-enhancing speaking behaviors, and modifying the feelings, beliefs, and emotions that accompany stuttering. These three components are addressed currently in the course of a client's stuttering therapy.

Managing Moments of Stuttering

This segment of therapy is about empowerment. Most who stutter feel that stuttering "happens to them"; they are its victim and feel helpless to change anything about it. It is unfortunate that we too frequently discard old ideas in favor of new ideas and innovations. Often, there are valuable and effective elements in the old ways that are dismissed. There is far too much value in Van Riper's Traditional Approach (Van Riper & Erickson, 1996) to therapy (stuttering modification) to dismiss it, just because it is not in vogue. The salvageable elements of the approach include teaching the client to objectively identify the core and secondary characteristics of his stuttering, learning how to modify it, and using the client's ability to predict stuttering moments to his advantage.

It is important to ensure that clients have an understanding of the complexity of speaking; an explanation of the anatomy and physiology of the normal process of speaking is a first step in educating the client in understanding how speech is produced. This also establishes a vocabulary that will aid the client's understanding of therapy and his stuttering. A simplified, functional discussion of the components of respiration, phonation, and articulation form the basis of discovering how the client's stuttering differs from normal speech production. Labeling anatomical features, understanding the underlying processes of breathing and speaking, and identifying stuttering behaviors educate the client and make him more knowledgeable of his stuttering. The language that is used and the tone of the discussion subtly transforms stuttering into an *objective*, rather than an *emotional* topic.

Clinical Insight: We typically view *emotions* and *logic* as polar opposites on a continuum. A person may be thought of as "too emotional" if they appear to make decisions primarily based upon their feelings. Others might be thought of as being "too logical" and criticized for not taking the feelings of others into consideration in their decision making process. In dealing with emotions relating to stuttering we attempt to change the client's perspective and focus on the objective aspects of his stuttering behaviors. Instead of the client characterizing a disfluent moment as being "bad" (an emotional label), we draw attention to the physical attributes of the stutter by identifying the type of disfluency (repetition, block, prolongation), the length of time it lasted, and where it occurred anatomically. Attending to these objective parameters draws the client from an emotional to a logical analysis of the event. Relatedly, the objective terms the clinician uses to talk about stuttering also influences the client's perspective. Stuttering becomes a "thing"; an animate object with tangible parameters. The subtle shift enables the client to loosen the emotional hold his stuttering has on him and better deal with the tangible behavioral characteristics.

An initial task is for the client to be able to identify the characteristics of his stuttering. This information later will be used to modify the disfluent behaviors. The observable characteristics include the type of disfluency (repetition, prolongation, or block), areas of tension, and the normal speech processes that were disrupted in the moment of stuttering. Other features to educate the client include the estimated length of the disfluency and the secondary characteristics that accompanied stuttered moments. For some clients, this is a painful process; for others it is an awakening. The emotional pain stems from confronting a long-standing, undesirable issue that denial has driven into a more comfortable place in the mind. Discussing stuttering, listening to audio recordings, watching videos of stuttering, or looking into a mirror shine a spotlight on the realities of the client's problem. Clients react in a variety of ways, ranging from withdrawing to acting out. The clinician needs to be aware and respond appropriately to the client's reactions, being sensitive and supporting, yet directive enough to lead the client to the desired objective.

Another underlying theme of therapy is that of responsibility. It is desirable for the language used to discuss the characteristics of stuttering to imply that the client is responsible for and can control these behaviors. For example, the clinician might point out, "I see that when you make a /p/ sound you start out with too much tension in your lips just before you are about to make the sound. That almost always results in your stuttering block." This identifies the client as being responsible for the behavior that resulted in his stuttering, rather than being a victim of a mysterious force. Many clients are reluctant to be held accountable for their stuttering, but in truth, along with the responsibility for stuttering comes the empowerment to change and control it. The speech techniques (stuttering modification and fluency shaping) become the tools to effect fluency and speaking confidence. But it is only through making the stuttering *their own* that the client is empowered to change it.

Most adults who stutter have a fairly habituated pattern of stuttering. By observing the patterns of the client's stuttering, the clinician identifies specific features of the stuttering to attack. One common feature is struggle: the extra effort the client uses to free himself or break away from a block. Struggle is related to one of the ironies of stuttering—the harder the client tries to force his way through a block, the harder the stutter becomes. It seems to be human nature to use more physical force when we meet obstacles. When you encounter difficulty unscrewing a cap from a jar, what do you do? Try harder! In stuttering, what is required though is easing up and letting the block slowly escape. In a way it is like "Chinese finger traps," the more effort you expend trying to pull your fingers out, the more entrapped you become. The secret, of course, is to work in opposition to your common sense, and use less effort pulling instead of more. The person who stutters must learn to "stutter smarter"; instead of pushing through a block, learning to slowly release it instead. Van Riper's pull-out technique is an example of this. Allow the client to have a block, and then demonstrate how he can slide out of it by reducing his muscular effort. With practice, clients can use this technique on each word and nearly avoid difficult blocks all together. Although pull-outs and other stuttering modification techniques are not meant to be the end product of therapy (we do not intend for the client's speech to sound like this at the termination of therapy), it does represent an effective means of modifying and controlling disfluencies. With time and a great deal of further practice, the duration of the pull-out can be made shorter and shorter. As clients gain control of their stuttering they become less anxious about speaking. This in turn triggers the less muscular tension and that results in less stuttering.

Other stuttering modification techniques include syllable stretching and easy starts. Syllable stretches require the client to intentionally prolong vowel sounds in words. This gives the speech a very artificial, stretched quality which sounds as though the speaker may have a muscular impairment, such as cerebral palsy or is intoxicated. Clients usually do not perceive this to be desirable, but it does serve as another tool to control stuttering. In the end, its gaining control of stuttering that is the critical skill.

Most stuttering occurs just as speech is initiated. Blocks at the level of the vocal folds are easily identified as no air is flowing out; it sounds and feels like the client is holding their breath or trying to lift a heavy object. Returning to our speech anatomy and physiology lesson, the vocal folds are adducted and do not allow air to be exhaled. The vocal folds are so tense it is nearly impossible for them to vibrate if exhalation were to start. Again, as a stuttering modification approach, easy starts serve to gradually release the tension on the vocal folds, allowing the client to "slide out" of the block. Employing this technique preventively before a block begins is even better. This is discussed as a fluency-shaping approach because it is a technique more akin to normal speaking than modifying stuttering.

Speech techniques to change stuttering behaviors empower the client to gain control of his stuttering when he is already in a stuttering block. This is a valuable and reassuring tool, something like an AAA card; when your car breaks down, you have a support plan and know just what to do. When speech fluency breaks down, the client now too has a lifeline. Again, the client has the responsibility to do something about his disfluencies, and the skills to work through disfluencies are such a lifeline.

Fluency-Enhancing Speaking Behaviors

This therapy approach deals with relearning a manner of speech production which is more compatible with natural speech fluency. Anxiety about speaking and stuttering often results in a client overcompensating in his attempt not to stutter. These overcompensations alter elements of an otherwise easy, natural speaking process by distorting one or more aspects of respiration, phonation, or articulation. Like other fluency shaping approaches in stuttering therapy, fluency-enhancing speaking behaviors emphasize and exaggerate the normal functions of breathing, voicing, and producing sounds.

We start by noting the processes of the client's habitual stuttering pattern which deviate from normal and then match the appropriate fluency-enhancing techniques to them. This approach emphasizes normal speech production rather than focusing on fixing stuttering. However, both approaches may have value for any specific client. For some clients, usually teens who do not relish dealing with their stuttering, focusing on aspects of speaking normally can be more palatable.

Respiration

There are two common breathing abnormalities in stuttering—inadequate breath support (running out of breath) and laryngeal blocking. Inadequate breath support is often the result of having expended too much air in struggling with disfluencies. From one perspective, the motor program that coordinates articulation and breathing is disrupted by the stuttering. The speaker's attempts to continue speaking are foiled because the original program is no longer adequate and fails to compensate for the excessive exhaled breath due to stuttering. In an attempt to "patch up" the speech motor program "on the fly," the speaker finds him- or herself out of air with still more words to say. The result is a forceful, strained attempt to squeeze out the remaining words on what little breath is left. This is somewhat analogous to slipping and trying to prevent yourself from falling while walking on an icy sidewalk. We have a motor plan for walking, but as we begin to slip we make rapid adjustments to the plan as necessitated by trying not to fall. The result is usually an awkward display of rapid movement which consumes energy inefficiently.

Laryngeal blocks occlude the flow of exhaled air to the degree that there is no air flowing or intermittent airflow; either situation being inadequate to support sustained phonation. Information and instruction on breathing (for respiration) and breathing for speech can be used to effectively address these problems. Instruction is provided to the client on the patterns of inhalation and exhalation components of restful breathing. Respiration for speech differs in that the inspiration phase is more rapid and the exhalation stage prolonged because we use the exhaled air for speaking.

Figure 3–2 displays a point at which inspiration ends and expiration begins. The client should be instructed to inhale and exhale, indentifying the moment at which the change

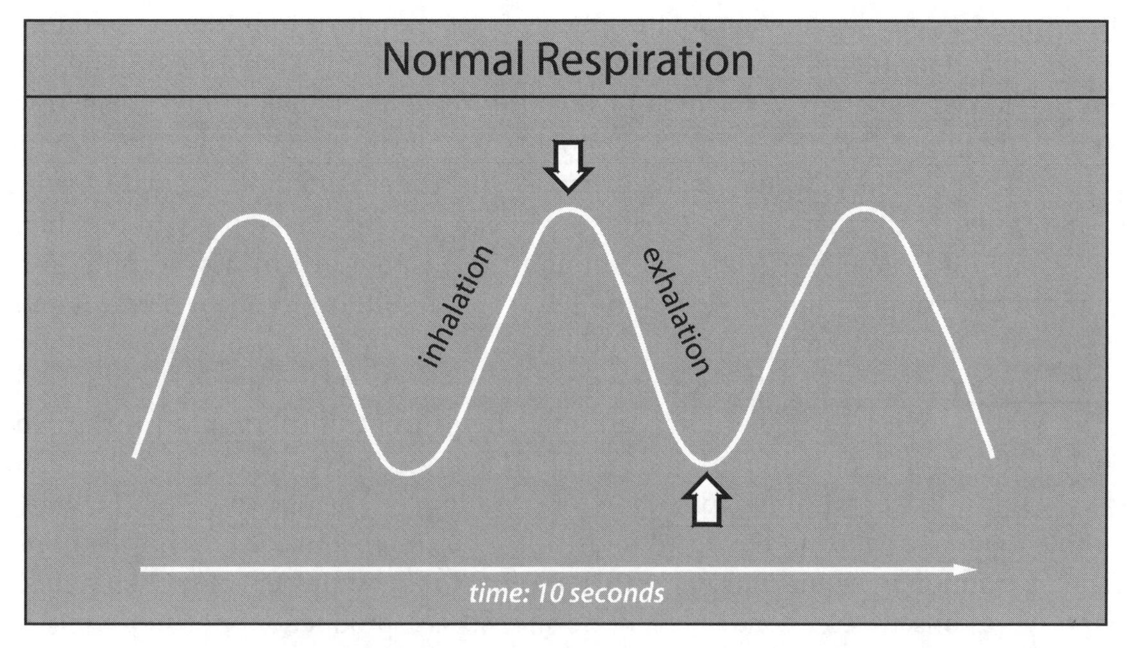

Figure 3–2. Respiration for breathing.

occurs. The vocal folds remain apart during both stages to allow for the free flow of air, in and out. For phonation, the vocal folds adduct very soon after the exhalation phase begins. The critical issue in stuttering, however, is the onset of voicing. Often, abnormal breathing patterns for speech are more a reflection of the client's attempts to doctor his disrupted speech program as a result of disfluencies. Abnormal breathing patterns may be a function of excessive anxiety as well. A discussion of normal speech breathing can benefit the patient in that it aids his awareness of when and how his aberrant breathing differs from normal. The element of initiating voicing is discussed next.

Inhalation is managed by expanding the volume of the thorax. This creates a negative air pressure (relative to the speaker's environment) or vacuum; this causes air to flow into the lungs. Thoracic volume can be increased either be moving the ribs upward and outward or by contracting the diaphragm. Have the client stand with his back to a wall in the treatment room and place one hand on his chest and the other on his belly. When he breathes, one of the hands will move. Movement of the hand on the chest is indicative of thoracic breathing and movement of the hand on the belly indicates diaphragmatic breathing. Usually, clients are thoracic breathers. Thoracic breathing may be affected more by the tension related to anxiety as it contracts the thoracic muscles and restricts movements for breathing. However, changing to diaphragmatic breathing is not as easy as it might appear. A thoracic breather has a very strong habit pattern established, having breathed in this manner literally hundreds of thousands of times unconsciously. However, discussing these two breathing styles may still be of value in educating the person who stutters about aspects of their speech and normal speech production.

Phonation

With respiration problems set aside, the client's focus may turn to initiating phonation. Many who stutter attempt to begin the voicing segment of speaking too abruptly. There is a rapid, forced initiation of voicing in which the vocal folds are jammed together with such force that they cannot vibrate. This condition usually results from the client's anxiety that he will not be able to speak. Again, ironically, the client's attempts to circumnavigate this situation actually increase the likelihood of its occurrence. Seemingly in an attempt to overcome and overpower stuttering through the element of surprise, a rapid, forced attempt at phonation usually leads to the inevitable result: a laryngeal block. Remarkably, there appears to be little learning from these failed attempts; people who stutter use this strategy repeated, and with the same undesirable result over and over again.

The Vocal Onset technique (discussed later) helps to begin phonation with greater ease. As exhalation begins, the client is instructed to bring the vocal folds together, slowly and very softly, like an airplane coming in for a landing on the runway. Slightly more air is exhaled before adducting the vocal folds. Once voicing begins, it is continued briefly before articulation is begun. Talking in this manner takes on the feel of speaking in slow motion. Vocal onset focuses on aspects of normal speech production, not stuttering, so it is considered a fluency enhancing technique. Clients learn to phonate for speech in a new way; one more compatible with fluency.

Some who stutter speak inappropriately loudly. Physiologically, loudness results in greater excursion of the vocal folds during phonation as they abduct. Overdriving the system in this way is unnecessary and increases the frequency of disfluencies. Excessive loudness may be a function of anxiety or the client's belief that communication partners are not listening to him; he may feel ineffective as a communicator. Either way, socially appropriate loudness or speaking softly serve to enhance fluency.

Articulation

Having accomplished the respiration and phonation components of fluent speech production, attention turns to articulation. Some clients appear to use excessive muscular effort in articulating sounds. Others exhibit a sloppy or mushy quality in their articulation. It may be that some people who stutter also have muscular coordination difficulties that affect their articulation. The misarticulations are distortions rather than substitutions or omissions of sounds. Although a relatively small subset of those adults who stutter, poorer articulation abilities may further complicate or be a contributing factor to their stuttering difficulties. For this group, slowing their speaking rate may enable them to articulate more accurately. We see that slowing speaking rate has a beneficial effect for almost everyone who stutters but, practically it is difficult to maintain. Nonetheless, having the client slow his rate and focus on articulating more crisply draws significantly more attention to the process of speaking. The client should feel like he is speaking purposefully, rather than spontaneously.

Articulation also comes into play in stuttering when clients use excessive muscular effort in sound production. This too is a result of nervousness and fear of stuttering. The forceful articulations represent the client's attempts to avoid stuttering by overpowering it. Forceful articulation attempts are often accompanied by rapid speaking rate. This combination significantly increases the risk of stuttering. A speaking technique used to address forceful articulation is called a *Light Articulatory Contact* or Light Contacts. As we move to articulate sounds, parts of the oral anatomy come into contact as the means of producing a specific sound. For example, in making the /p/ sound, the upper and lower lips make contact. For the /t/ sound, the tip of the tongue contacts the alveolar ridge. The muscular effort required to make the contact is extremely slight. The Light Contact Technique focuses the client's attention to utilizing the minimal amount of pressure when structures come into contact to produce a sound. Again, speaking becomes a series of volitionally connected motor movements, rather than the spontaneous outpouring of speech. Speaking rate is slowed to aid the client in monitoring the soft, gentle contact of the articulators.

Other Fluency-Enhancing Speaking Techniques

Almost universally, a slower speaking rate dramatically effects a reduction or elimination of stuttering. Although very simple, at the same time it can be exceedingly difficult to maintain. Speaking rate is a reflection of social and cultural norms; it is also indicative

Clinic Perspectives: It has been observed that when the process of speaking is made easier, even by one element, fluency usually improves. Having the client whisper (removing the element of voicing) or having him sing (removing the elements of generating speech and generating intonation/melody) are well known to significantly reduce the frequency of stuttering.

A majority of adult clients who stutter want their speech to "just come out." What is required in therapy is speaking in a "nonspontaneous" way, making each sound in a deliberate, disciplined fashion. It is easy to appreciate the desire for speech to be natural and carefree, being able to go quickly and effortlessly from thought to utterance. However, in the initial stages of speech therapy for those who stutter, there are no shortcuts. A key ingredient in effective therapy requires speaking to be a purposeful act; not spontaneous.

of the speaker's emotional state. Our rate slows when we do not feel well or when we are tired; it increases to reflect excitement or nervousness. It can be difficult to speak quickly when we are ill; it just does not seem to fit. Conversely, it is hard to speak slowly when we are excited greeting a good friend we have not seen in a long time. When an emotion is aroused (such as when being anxious about stuttering), the perception of one's own rate becomes exaggerated. Asked to speak slowly when excited, the perception of how slow this new rate actually is becomes distorted; it feels V-E-R-Y slow and unnatural because it seems not to match the emotional state. In reality it may be well within a range of normal, but it seems peculiar to the speaker, and peculiar is commonly thought to be "bad."

Other reasons to speak slowly (other than improved fluency) may need to be explored with the client to motivate him to slow his speaking rate. One approach is that of being an effective communicator. Many people who stutter feel that they are ineffective communicators, and thus this approach will likely have an appeal to the client. On the surface, the role of a good communicator is to provide information to his listener. But, at a slightly deeper level, to be effective, the communicator must additionally take responsibility for the listener to understand the message, not just hear it. Communication is not merely "dumping" or "throwing" information at the listener; it needs to be understood. Thus, to communicate effectively, the speaker must also create optimal conditions to promote the listener's understanding of the message. One such condition is to present the information at a speaking rate that enables the listener to process and understand what is said.

A neighbor was once teaching her young son to cross the street safely. Her instruction was, "Look both ways before you cross." Her son did exactly what his mother requested. He stood on the sidewalk, his head snapped to the right, then quickly snapped to the left, and he then started the cross the street. However, he moved his head back and forth so quickly that he didn't take the time for the "picture" to register—he didn't actually see anything, he just moved his head to the right and to the left—his token gesture of "looking both ways." When a speaker talks too quickly, there frequently isn't time to really think about what he is saying, the used car salesman technique. A good communicator who wants the listener to understand what he is saying must deliver his message in a way that allows time to process it. One key ingredient of communicating effectively is speaking slowly, and deliberately. And for the person who stutters, there is also a boost to their fluency.

Working with Emotions: Anxiety, Fear, Negative Past Experiences

Fears and Anxiety

Fears and anxiety about speaking are common among people who stutter. Fear is a deeply ingrained bodily response to danger; it is fundamental to preserving life. People need to be cautious and avoid serious dangers to survive. Anxiety is related to fear; it is a general feeling of apprehension, a premonition of impending danger. An intense, excessive fear of an activity, object, or situation is known as a phobia. With phobias, the fear is out of proportion to the actual physical danger at hand. Phobias cause a person to take action or make alterations to avoid perceived physical or psychological dangers. For some who stutter, their phobia relates to speaking in social contexts. Their fear is out of proportion to the actual danger.

The Role of Fear and Anxiety in Stuttering

Anxiety, fear, and phobias are an integral part of the problem of stuttering. Speaking phobias result in limiting or restricting activities in which patients are willing to participate. As a consequence, these avoidances and restrictions handicap their lives.

For those who stutter, patterned behaviors, negative thinking, and a belief system about speaking and stuttering emerge, which magnify to intensity of the problem. This way of thinking and the habitual behavior patterns that follow from it become internalized and the person who stutters begins to construct his life around his fears about speaking. He begins to form his self-concept around the inability to speak and the fear of being embarrassed.

Fear and anxiety can represent a bigger problem than the actual stuttering itself, as we see in cases of covert stuttering. These thought patterns and belief systems also contribute heavily to problem of relapse. The body's response to fear and anxiety blocks the client's ability to access the therapy targets, particularly during moments of stress. As a result, many who stutter stop speaking altogether, rather than risk stuttering uncontrollably.

The Body's Response to Fear

There are three consequences of fear: behavioral, cognitive, and physiologic. Behavioral symptoms are the actions that result from being fearful. When in a fearful state, behavioral symptoms may include things such as shakiness, throat clearing, and avoidances. Cognitive symptoms include less flexibility in thinking and greater difficulty with deeper thinking (the brain responds in a more reflexive way); our system becomes hypersensitive and there is greater selective focus on the feared stimulus. Physiologic symptoms include increased heart and respiration rates, and increased blood flow to large muscle groups and perspiring. These are the ways our body responds to fear, as in the "fight or flight" response. The body prepares for action by sending energy to large muscle groups to either fight or flee. This response poorly serves the act of speaking, which requires a high degree of intellect, fine motor movements, and great deal of coordination.

How the Response Is Elicited

The emotion of fear is elicited when an event or situation is perceived to be threatening. The person becomes aware on an impending physical or psychological danger, a threat to the ego or the person's sense of self. Two factors enhance the fear response: memories of past experiences and apprehension (the premonition of impending danger). Previous bad experiences in similar situations are stored vividly in memory. These emotional memories serve to accentuate the memory of the event or situation. Apprehension intensifies the sensitivity of systems that scan for danger; it sets them "on edge." Apprehension thereby heightens the impact of fear. For example, for the client who has difficulty saying his name, apprehension is generated while waiting as people take their turn introducing themselves going around the table at a meeting. The tension grows step by step as the client's turn to say his name comes closer and closer. The memory of past failures (and the consequences of everyone laughing, commenting, and snickering that the speaker doesn't even know his own name) is brought to mind in a split second. Many can feel their heart pounding in anticipation and fear. The response may be initiated when the group leader invites everyone to introduce themselves as the meeting is brought to order. For some, the apprehension begins leaving their office to attend the meeting. For yet others, the apprehension begins weeks earlier when the meeting is scheduled. The response begins when the person realizes that a dangerous situation has arisen. The fear response is elicited automatically, and although it cannot be extinguished, clients can learn how to mediate it with the clinician's help. The body's response to fear, a "call to action," is instantly summoned. This primitive reflex, however, is not particularly helpful in circumstances that are not actually life threatening, like the fear of speaking. Both fighting and fleeing involve activation of large muscle groups, increasing heart and respiration rates. Mediation of higher cerebral thinking is diminished. These bodily reactions are exactly the opposite of what is required to effectively manage fluency. The "fight or flight" response is rooted very deeply in our genetics and cannot be extinguished. Our work then becomes a matter of learning to mediate our reactions, minimizing their impact on speech disfluency.

Treating Fears and Anxiety

The treatment paradigm to manage the fear response is to combat it mentally. Remember, it is unrealistic to expect the reflex to go away; it is primitive and still critical to our survival. But one general approach is to begin by making the feared events more tangible and objective. The approach begins by becoming more knowledgeable of the symptoms of our fear by increasing cognitive awareness. It is human nature to avoid fears. But to overcome them, one must first become more knowledgeable about them, knowledgeable of both the bodily feelings and the object of the fears.

There are three components of fear to learn more about: (1) how the body specifically responds to fear, (2) evaluating the degree of the fear response, and (3) building more tolerance for the fear.

1. Clinicians should help the client explore the ways in which their body is affected by fear. The body's response to fear can serve as a framework to guide the client's exploration. The more detailed the exploration, the richer and more complete the understanding, and the more helpful it will prove to be. This knowledge can be used to add rationality to the sensation of fear and diminish the emotions. Once the client understands what is happening, why his heart is pounding, why his hands are shaking, and why he is feeling "butterflies" in his stomach, he can reassure himself with thoughts such as, "That's just my body responding to being nervous; so my body is working just fine! It will be okay."
2. Fear is based on perception and, as such, can be measured on a perceptual scale. Have the patient assess the level of his or her fear relative to the extremes on a continuum. A 10-point scale is commonly used with "10" signifying an immediate, unstoppable, life-threatening event (such as just about to be struck down and killed by a bus) and "1" defining a state of relaxation near sleep. The scale helps the patient cognitively evaluate, critically compare, and communicate the status of their mental and bodily response to fear. Instead of fleeing, they are using their intellect to analyze and grade their emotional fear response.
3. The intent is not to extinguish the fear, but to be able to better tolerate it so that the fear reflex is not set off to the 10 level, but is gauged and responded to at the appropriate level. This may be approached by listening to the messages you send to yourself in fearful situations. These messages may not be words, but rather impulses. An initial step is to listen for that impulse, then translate it into words. Being able to articulate the messages is an important initial step toward modifying and changing the message, to allow the patient to respond differently and appropriately for the situation.

At best, the fears and anxieties associated with stuttering can be better managed; it is not reasonable to think they can be easily extinguished, but they can diminish over time as less fear is associated with speaking. It is difficult for many people who stutter to comprehend that people who don't stutter are the least bit anxious or fearful of public speaking. Learning how to mediate the process by which fear and anxiety is elicited and communicated throughout the body can be an effective means of managing the response, enabling the client to function appropriately.

Reactions to stuttering and the feelings they evoke represent one of the biggest obstacles in stuttering therapy. People who stutter have strong feelings about their stuttering, and those feelings are not positive ones. Most people who stutter develop anxiety, nervousness, and apprehension about speaking as they fear the repetition of episodes of stuttering they have learned arise uncontrollably. The emotions that surround stuttering greatly complicate therapy. These affective characteristics of stuttering diminish the client's cognitive control and awareness of speaking; they interfere with the ability to think clearly and objectively, thereby lessening the likelihood of speaking fluently.

As previously discussed, anxiety leads to increased muscle tension (usually in the articulators and vocal folds) and decreased cognitive awareness. Additionally, people have a propensity to increase speaking rate when nervous. In response to the fear of stuttering, clients are prone to trying to overpower stuttering moments, which results in greater struggle behaviors. Reversing these emotional reflexes helps to lessen them as obstacles to therapy.

There are several other approaches to reduce the effects of fear and anxiety; they include decreasing the fear of stuttering, utilizing compensations in the speaking process, and rebuilding the client's self-concept as a communicator. As everyone knows, fear seemingly has the ability to take over instantly when it is elicited. Emotions overtake rational thoughts and the client feels as though he is spiraling out of control. The sight of a spider or the squealing brakes of a car as you cross the street send ripples of emotion through the brain and throughout the body. The physical reactions are immediate, reflexive, and strong; they are both learned and instinctive.

There is much to be learned from approaches used to deal with phobias; working through a hierarchy of proximity to the feared stimulus, developing a more objective awareness, and building a rational knowledge base are each avenues which may be fruitful. However, an understanding of the fear itself is an important starting point for the clinician. In stuttering, the fear is not of physical harm, but emotional harm. So the goal is essentially ego protection, yet the emotions and bodily responses are the same as those elicited when physical harm is at risk. Through our senses, the brain is alerted to a potential danger. Neurochemicals are released in the brain by the amygdala that trigger the body's emergency response mechanisms (the "flight or fight response"). Some fear triggers appear to be inherited or innate, whereas others are learned. For example, rabbits appear to be instinctively fearful of hawks and other birds of prey; their life (and the lives of their offspring) depend on it. But infants are not inherently afraid of spiders or snakes; these fears are learned, usually from a parent or caretaker. Fear of stuttering is learned too; it is not instinctual. As the person who stutters learns from the reaction of others that something is "wrong" with the way he speaks, fears develop that incidents of stuttering will occur again, which again will lead to ridicule by others. The fear causes muscle tension, increased speaking rate, and more stuttering occurs, seemingly out of the speaker's control. Attempts to overpower stuttering moments lead to more physical tension and struggle, making the stuttering more frequent and more overt. The fear grows, becomes more pronounced, and is generalized to more speaking situations. The client becomes increasingly aware and scans for impending speaking situations which may elicit his undesirable stuttering. Although "flight" (avoidance) from these situations provides temporary relief, it only serves to build and intensify the fear, thereby increasing its perceived validity and power. These factors serve to intensify the fear and fuel anxiety, which increase the likelihood of more and more stuttering. The client feels victimized and helpless to do anything about his stuttering. He feels out of control.

Clients who stutter are sometimes resistant to speaking or trying to communicate. To a large degree their fears and anxiety shape their personality and cause them to make decisions based on their stuttering, like deciding what to order at a restaurant based on what they can say. Reversing this is not a small undertaking. Years in the making, these beliefs become etched in the psyche of the individual; to the point where making any change to it, even one that results in greater fluency, can be extremely difficult.

Part of the strategy to break down these obstacles is to transform the emotionally loaded behaviors into objectively based characteristics in the process of defusing them. We can start by educating the client about stuttering; teaching him factual data and learning about the different types of disfluencies, and which ones are characteristic of the client's own stuttering. This discussion is not a judgment of the client's worth, but an objective inventory of the characteristics of his stuttering. It may be useful to begin by identifying the characteristics of someone else's stuttering by watching a video of another person stuttering. The client and clinician work together to label the stuttering behaviors observed. Later, the client is asked to identify the types of stuttering that characterize his speech; watching a video or audio recording may be helpful, but at first may be too great a confrontation for the client.

Ask the client to estimate the length of time a disfluency lasts. Verify his perception with a stopwatch. It is not uncommon for the client to overestimate (and sometimes grossly overestimate!) the duration of a stutter. In part, this reflects the client's discomfort with his stuttering. When the stuttering makes the client uncomfortable, his mind exaggerates the perception of its duration. Time seems to stand still when stuttering and the client may feel as though his stuttering block lasted "forever." Again, this is an attempt to help the client gather objective information about his stuttering.

Following a brief review of the basic anatomy and physiology of the speaking process, ask the client what he does differently when he stutters. Is exhalation cut off? Are the vocal folds too tense to vibrate to produce voice? Is there appropriate (not excessive) tension in the lips, tongue, and other articulators during disfluent moments? The intent is for the client to be able to describe his stuttering in objective terms and discuss it as an intellectual, rather than emotional, experience.

It is important to use language that subtly implies that the client is responsible for these differences; this is the "language of empowerment." It is not his fault that he stutters; but it is his responsibility to manage it. If he is responsible for doing it incorrectly, he should be responsible (and therefore empowered) to change his behavior. Specific speaking techniques or targets will be employed to help in this process of taking command of his speech.

It also is important to help the client become less sensitive to his stuttering and more accepting of himself as a person who stutters. Sizable efforts are usually put forth by clients to guard against disclosing themselves as a person who stutters. Thus, thoughts of volunteering such information or "advertising" their stuttering are all but unthinkable from a client's perspective, and most clients recoil even from discussing the idea. Nonetheless, it is a worthwhile venture to pursue in therapy, and one of a few things that take the "sting" out of stuttering. Some clients retort that others already know they stutter, so telling them they stutter would be redundant. But there is a subtle difference between someone observing the stuttering and being told about it. For example, when you meet someone in a wheelchair with a physical disability, it is considered socially inappropriate to ask what's wrong with their legs. But if the wheelchair-bound person is first to bring up his disability, it is more acceptable to discuss his situation. Acknowledging what is obvious seemingly removes the taboo of having a conversation about it and takes away the tension. Ironically, it seems to disarm the topic as a source of ridicule and evokes gestures of support and sincere interest in the person who stutters. Yet, it is very hard for the client who stutters to do that, as past experiences of derision are difficult to overcome. This represents a huge risk and it can take a long time to convince a client of the merit. However, once accomplished, clients report that they are at far greater ease about stuttering; their secret has come out, but on their own terms.

Another issue in addressing the emotional bases of stuttering has to do with the cause of stuttering. The cause of stuttering has long been a mystery and the subject of a great deal of unfortunate speculation. Although science continues to search for a cause, misinformation and half-truths about the etiology of stuttering persist. Stuttering, as an intellectual topic, is usually very intriguing to people. Why do people who stutter not stutter when they sing or talk by themselves when alone? Why does stuttering disappear when speaking to the beat of a metronome or when the client cannot hear themselves talk? But without knowing factual information about stuttering, the client is unable to discuss his stuttering when an opportunity presents itself. Helping the client to script an explanation of stuttering enables him to turn a critical remark about his stuttering into the topic of an intellectual conversation. The client becomes the source of knowledge and information about stuttering, turning a heckler into a conversational partner. People usually credit others who are afflicted with a disorder to have special knowledge about it. Arming the client with a script can serve to transform ridicule into having a friendly, interesting conversation. "Oh, that's just my stutter. Did you know that four times as many men stutter as women, and that 80% of children who stutter recover? Stuttering tends to run in families, but no one else in my family stutters." A conversation of this nature elevates the communication exchange and places the client in a respected position as "educator", rather than a victim of a mysterious disability. The more facts that are known, the more intriguing the conversation becomes, even if the speech is stuttered.

The ability to manage one's feelings and emotions is a long-term prospect that can take considerable time, persistence, trust, and guidance to achieve. It may always be a struggle. However, these very components make stuttering the challenging problem it is. Changing the way a person thinks alters his behavior. This is particularly true of stuttering. Being able to modify and change the client's perceptions of his or her stuttering is likely the single most important factor in developing a successful long-term result.

Working With Covert Stuttering

Case Profile

Practically no one knows that Jeff stutters. His parents were a little concerned about his speech in elementary school, but now they rarely notice anything different about the way he talks; they feel lucky that Jeff was one of the lucky ones who "outgrew" their stuttering. Jeff does pause a lot when speaking, but who doesn't? It's just his speaking style. Maybe he's thinking of the right word or a something funny to say about the situation, but stutter? No way.

Jeff sometimes goes to great lengths to keep people from knowing that he stutters. He frequently changes words; he misses classes when he has to do a presentation; and orders foods that are easier for him to say. He's pretty talkative and likes to hang out with everyone. Most others, including his parents, have no idea of the planning and "mental gymnastics" that Jeff goes through trying to hide his stuttering. He constantly scans the environment for "dangers" in which he might stutter. He has many strategies to use to get out of speaking situations and an encyclopedia of excuses and explanations about his minor speech "hiccups." Jeff rarely allows himself to stutter and he is very careful never to talk about it or acknowledge it with others. Although no one sees him stutter, his life is governed by the fear that his secret will be exposed.

When the penalties for stuttering are strong they can cause the person to take extreme measures to conceal it, rather than risk exposing it. This is the basis of covert stuttering. Covert stuttering is perhaps a more challenging problem for the clinician because it is "invisible"; and working with a problem that cannot be seen or heard complicates treating it. It might be argued that covert stuttering is actually more severe than those whose stuttering is characterized by frequent overt disfluencies, even though it does not necessarily appear so on severity rating scales. With covert stuttering, the penalties—the embarrassment, shame, guilt—are so great that the person is not willing to risk being exposed. Those who stutter overtly experience the same emotions, fears, and anxieties about their stuttering, but they cannot inhibit their stuttering from coming out. Rather than risk stuttering, individuals who stutter covertly choose to pause, switch words, or, in some cases, do not speak at all. They do not allow themselves to stutter and often go to very great lengths not to reveal their stuttering and to ensure that no one knows. For example, an acquaintance who stutters covertly went back through all her family's home videos of herself as a child and edited out all of the scenes that she felt revealed her disfluencies. Word avoidances (switching a word perceived to be troublesome for another word) or electing not to speak at all are behaviors common in covert stuttering. However, the extreme measures to which some have resorted demonstrate the level of fear and strength of the emotions generated by their stuttering. Usually, the disfluencies of those who stutter covertly tend to be much milder, enabling them to get away without being detected as a person who stutters, masquerading as a fluent speaker.

It is important to understand how the person who stutters thinks about their stuttering. The ends they are willing to employ to try to conceal it help indicate which normal sounding speech is likely stuttering being covered up. Generally, severity ratings of covert stutterers tend to be categorized as mild or very mild; in some cases, there are no disfluencies to count! However, this does not mean that the handicapping effects of their problem are any less than those of overt stutterers. Hiding stuttering is accomplished by a variety of means. One common trick is to substitute words, using a word the client is confident he can say for one that he fears he will stutter. Word substitutions often complicate attempts to formulate the message that was intended. Sometimes branching to other (substituted) words clouds the message and confuses the listener. Try saying a few sentences and changing every third word that you had planned to say. Notice how much mental effort is spent in word selection—better open up the thesaurus! In the process, note how your sentences sort of weave in, out and around your intended thought stream. Most people find this mentally exhausting; but apparently better than stuttering! One clue in determining if the client is substituting words is to compare their fluency while reading aloud with their speech in conversation. Clients who substitute usually demonstrate more disfluencies in reading than in spontaneous conversation, because attempts to substitute words are obvious when reading from a designated passage.

Another strategy is using frequent pauses while speaking. Clients pause prior to saying a word, waiting for the feeling that "it's okay now" before proceeding. They do not allow themselves to stutter. They sometimes add to the deception by acting as if they are trying to think of just the right word to say or that they are contemplating how to better express their ideas. This is a strategy sometimes observed in bilingual clients speaking in their nonnative language. Still others avoid stuttering by not talking at all or talking very little; they are often thought of as being shy or just a person who doesn't talk much. Sometimes, their communication consists primarily of making offhand comments following someone else's lead.

Covert stutterers often structure their world around their stuttering. For example, at a restaurant they might order what they can say instead of what they want, or not answer questions in class even when they know the answer, or drive over to someone's house instead of calling them on the phone. In the classroom, children often are called on to read passages aloud to the entire class. Teachers usually call on students in a predictable order, such as from the front to the back of each row. One student who stuttered that when called on to read, dropped a pencil on the floor, bent down and picked it up, and then stabbed it through his hand so he would have to be taken to the school nurse, all so that he wouldn't have to read aloud. The pain of running the pencil through his hand outweighed the embarrassment of stuttering in front of his classmates.

The first part of the clinician's challenge is to encourage the client to reveal this stuttering, to let the stuttering out for the world to see and hear. This usually is no small feat. Most covert clients find this confrontation overwhelming. Because they can adeptly negotiate around their stuttering, they often feel that disclosure is not necessary, enabling their secret to be maintained. In that sense, it is human nature to avoid pain and discomfort. But that is not the path toward overcoming it.

Another objection often raised by clients is the belief that allowing their stutter to come out makes it seem like their stuttering is getting worse. If you were to count the number of disfluencies as the measure of severity, they would be absolutely correct. But, in reality, letting stuttering out (acknowledging it) is a huge step in the longer process of reducing the severity and the handicaps it causes. This is a very positive beginning.

Be prepared for the client's discomfort to be expressed in various ways. Patients have actually stood up and left the room; a few have opted to quit therapy, some have cried, and some have gotten angry, all of which may be seen as affirmative reactions toward overcoming this hurdle in their therapy. For some, it's a catharsis in which years of pent up emotions are finally released, sometimes in an awkward, uncontrolled manner.

Therapy Approaches for Covert Stuttering

An overall goal in therapy for covert stuttering is for the client to get his or her stuttering out in the open, revealing and acknowledging it to others. There is no formula or simple approach that works for everyone, so finding the path for any particular client is part of the art of stuttering therapy. Most clients do not want to let their secret out; it is human nature not to want to reveal our flaws. Complicating the issue with mild stuttering is that clients feel they can "get away" with not having to disclose that they stutter. But, at its root, that deception is a lie. The lie forms the foundation for a pattern of lies required in the attempt to maintain the original deception. For example, some people who stutter who have difficulty saying their name have used a different name when introducing themselves to a stranger. They then need to maintain their "new identity" so it will not seem strange that they lied about their name in the first place. This web can become quite complicated and represents the penalty or handicap trying to conceal stuttering can perpetuate. Covert stuttering affects persons who stutters in that they live with their deception and their subsequent need to be constantly on guard against circumstances in which their secret may be revealed.

Understand that the client perceives his stuttering to be a significant "defect" or personal flaw, one significant enough to need to hide and lie about it. Consequently, disclosing their secret is not a welcomed opportunity. For people who stutter, covertly and overtly alike, there is shame in stuttering and it is hard to overestimate the significance most place on it or, more accurately, place on hiding it. The longer the secret is maintained and left "unspoken," the stronger the importance of hiding it becomes.

There are subtle and some more direct approaches for the client to disclose his stuttering. Therapy might begin by having the client intentionally repeat the first words of an utterance in a very light, effortless fashion, "putting his stuttering out there," testing to see if anyone notices. Becoming comfortable and accepting a few, very mild, voluntary disfluencies can be a first step. Later requests will come for more pronounced, effortful disfluencies, more characteristic of the client's real stuttering.

What is hard for clients to appreciate is how much more significant and meaningful their stuttering is to them than it is to other people. It is hard for clients to understand the importance of the context as well. There is sort of an irony. When someone stutters and does not acknowledge it, others see it as humorous or as something to be ridiculed. But when a person who stutters does so openly and acknowledges it to others, the interpersonal dynamic changes. The stuttering that was previously the subject of ridicule can now become a topic of intellectual conversation; and to listeners, this usually evokes emotions of compassion or wanting to provide support and assistance. But the prior experiences of people who stutter do not enable them to predict the likelihood of this listener reaction. The client expects that, if he were to admit his stuttering, ridicule would result and his fear would be strengthened. He does not yet appreciate the subtlety of the difference that acknowledging his stuttering to the listener, getting ahead of his stutter, will make.

When a discussion of stuttering becomes an objective or intellectual topic, most who stutter are ill equipped to discuss it knowledgeably or confidently. Others are quick to assume that, when someone stutters, they must be a well-versed expert on it. As a conversational topic, most people are truly curious about stuttering. This creates the opportunity for the client to educate others about stuttering, which also disarms the ridicule. Additionally, it transforms the person from being perceived as a victim of the disorder to becoming an expert and source of knowledge and information. It therefore is prudent for clients to develop a script about stuttering to prepare them for their new role as educator. Developing and rehearsing the script about the causes of stuttering and other factual information also helps the person who stutters become better educated himself. But, more importantly, it also makes talking about stuttering easier.

When some clients are asked if they have told others that they stutter, they often respond by saying, "They already know just by listening to me. So I don't need to tell them!" Many clients who have offered this argument have gone on discover the difference this disclosure makes. It is not whether or not the listener knows about the stuttering as much as the circumstances by which they find out that makes the meaningful difference. Most clients discover that disclosing their stuttering puts *them* at ease as much or more than their listener. Sometimes people who stutter are invited to speak about their stuttering to classes at their school or at a university. After disclosing to the class that they stutter, their stuttering can magically disappear (or at least diminish greatly)! Often, once the secret is out, the anxiety behind it being uncovered disappears, making way for more natural fluency as the tension dissipates. Successful clients free themselves of the fear of others discovering that they stutter. Letting "the secret" affect daily decisions, no matter how fluent the client may be, is not the same as being free of stuttering. Covert stuttering, although seemingly only mildly troublesome to the observer, brings with it the same angst and other emotions as overt stuttering. But for the clinician, covert stuttering is usually a more challenging clinical case in therapy.

Determining a Starting Point for Therapy

There often are an overwhelming number of things to address in therapy, so determining a logical starting point can be confusing. One approach is to identify the symptoms and speech characteristics of the client's stuttering that contribute most to the perceived severity of the problem. For example, some clients struggle through each instance of stuttering persistently when they are disfluent. These struggle behaviors exaggerate the outward appearance of the severity of the problem. Consequently, a starting place for this client might be to reduce the struggle behaviors by working on stuttering modification techniques that will minimize or greatly reduce the struggle. In other cases, excessive use of starters or interjections results in speech that technically may be stutter-free, but is so disjointed that it draws unfavorable attention to the speaker and makes it hard to follow his thoughts. For this client, therapy might begin by eliminating interjections and establishing the habit of going directly to the feared word by using an appropriate fluency shaping technique. This serves to "clean up" the client's speech and develop a more empowered, confident style of speaking.

In designing a therapy plan for a client, begin by listing the speech symptoms of their overt speaking characteristics and other stuttering behaviors. Next, identify the two or three components that have the biggest impact on the problem. At the client's current level of functioning, determine which he is most capable of changing. This may be a good place to begin therapy because of the potential impact on stuttering severity and the client's demonstrated ability to change.

A component of therapy for all new clients is to understand the normal speech production process. With each new client, time is spent teaching the basic anatomy and physiology of respiration, phonation, and articulation. This establishes a vocabulary that facilitates communication throughout the course of treatment. It also provides clients with an understanding of the normal speaking process, from which they can discover how their stuttering behaviors differ. This initial step leads clients to identify the specific parameters of their stuttering and other behavioral speaking characteristics. This is Van Riper's "Identification" phase of stuttering therapy. Many clients respond so strongly and negatively to their stuttering they are not always cognizant of exactly what is happening. Starting by describing the behaviors that constitute their stuttering begins the process of objectifying stuttering in the client's mind. Shifting emotional reactions to objective, factual descriptions is an important aspect of therapy. The overarching objective of accepting stuttering and depersonalizing it is facilitated by viewing it as a behavior, rather than a personal imperfection.

> **Clinical Insight:** Stay focused. There are so many aspects of stuttering that may need to be addressed that it's easy to try to fix them all at once. It is important to construct a plan identifying a few important goals (or objectives) to be addressed in therapy. Stay focused on these goals or therapy will become scattered and less effective. Clients can also begin to feel that there is so much wrong with the way that they speak that they will not be able to be successful. Be sure the client is aware of the specific targets that his therapy is addressing and why you feel they are the most important aspects to be working on right now.

Therapy Techniques (Targets)

Therapy targets are selected to address the specific stuttering symptoms of the individual client's disfluencies; his blocks, repetitions, and prolongations. There also are targets that address the secondary characteristics and the client's thoughts and beliefs about his stuttering. Speech targets generally fall into two categories: fluency enhancing (speaking in a manner that facilitates fluency based on the normal speech processes) and stuttering management (modifying and controlling disfluencies). Some clients, particularly teens, resist talking about stuttering or trying to modify their stuttering as the confrontation is too great. As a result, selecting fluency-enhancing targets may be more palatable to the client as they do not deal directly with stuttering. Rather, they are perceived as steps leading directly toward their aspiration of speaking fluently in a manner based on normal speech production. For clients who present obstacles to the subject of stuttering, fluency-enhancement strategies may prove to be a more fruitful approach. A disadvantage of adhering exclusively to fluency enhancement is that the client would not be skilled in managing disfluencies when they occur. Typically, most treatment programs include both fluency-enhancement and stuttering-modifications techniques in a proportion based on the client's needs and willingness to use them.

Fluency-Enhancing Targets

Teaching normal aspects of speaking. The pattern and many speaking behaviors of people who stutter often contribute to a client's stuttering. One approach is to teach the client how to modify and change his stuttering; this is called the Stuttering-Modification Approach.

Another approach instructs the client to speak in different ways that enhance the likelihood that fluent speech will result. Components of this Fluency-Enhancing Approach are based on normal speech production. Instead of teaching the client how to change his stuttering, this approach instructs him to speak in a manner more compatible with fluency.

Slow Rate

Client Profile

Bill is very self-conscious about his stuttering and constantly fears that others will notice it and think poorly of him. His family and friends frequently suggest that he "just slow down a little" when he has difficulty speaking. But Bill never seems to be able to heed their advice. Because he is so anxious, sometimes he begins answering a question before his communication partner is finished asking it. He begins utterances very abruptly; his speech sounds like he is racing from one stuttering block to the next. People frequently ask him to repeat what he has said because it is often hard to understand what he said. Bill finds this very aggravating; having struggled to get his message out, he then needs to repeat it. This just sets the stage for even more disfluencies the second and third time. Speaking so rapidly, some sounds aren't articulated crisply and the rhythm of his speech also suffers as a result. When he is anxious his rate accelerates; he is conscious of it, but has real difficulty slowing it down. Most of these symptoms are nonexistent in speaking situations in which he is totally relaxed, like talking to his dog.

Rationale

Speaking is a very complex activity that integrates cognitive and mental functions with motor movements, allowing the individual to express his thoughts and ideas with meaning and emotion. The complex nature of this very rapid, highly coordinated activity is truly amazing. Any of a multitude of factors can serve to disrupt the smooth flow of speech: a momentary difficulty retrieving a word, an auditory or visual distraction, recognition of an incorrect syntactical construction, difficulty managing a strong emotion, or pushing the speaking process too quickly by hurrying.

Every person has an optimal speed at which he or she can speak, maintaining the precision and coordination of motor movements, integrated with all of the other components involved in communicating. Slowing the habitual speed of speaking slightly usually has many benefits for just about all speakers. A slower rate allows greater precision of movement and enhances oral motor coordination. It allows more time to put thoughts into words, the opportunity to select words which more accurately reflect the intended meaning, more time to appreciate the listener's perspective, et cetera. Furthermore, using slower rate is perceived as being more relaxed and is often associated with people perceived to be more important and more knowledgeable.

The clinician might explain to the patient, *"Most people who stutter are anxious about speaking and afraid that they will stutter again. These fears cause the rate at which you speak to increase. I've noticed that as your rate gets faster, the frequency of your stuttering increases too. Your natural reaction to your fears in this situation causes you to speak too rapidly. As a consequence, you need to compensate for this tendency by deliberately speaking at a very slow rate. I think you will see that it will have a significant effect on your speech fluency. At first it might sound too slow; but you will also note that you stutter much less. In time you won't need to speak quite this slowly; but at the beginning it usually works best to really exaggerate. Let's try to read this paragraph aloud, speaking as slowly as I am speaking to you right now."*

There is a point at which rate can be too slow. A very slow rate may give the impression that the speaker is ill or under the influence of alcohol, drugs or other conditions, or perhaps not too smart. People who stutter are generally quite sensitive to others' perceptions of them. Most clients feel uncomfortable initially using slow rate, fearing that listeners will think that something is wrong with them or that they are stupid. This feeling is accentuated by the person who stutters because his anxiety about speaking exaggerates and distorts his own perception of this new, slower rate. So a "slow normal" rate is targeted at which the client is obviously controlling his speaking rate well below his habitual rate. In time, clients become accustomed to speaking at a slow normal rate and the feelings that it is "different," and therefore "wrong," subside.

Some say that speaking at a slower rate adds 15 IQ points to others' perception of you! For the person who stutters, it also adds fluency. Considering speaking solely from a motor perspective; slowing down reduces the demands on the system, allowing more time for movement accuracy and coordination. For the person who stutters, finding the optimal speed (the speed at which movement is most accurate and disfluencies are not triggered) equates to the rate at which the system functions optimally. "Speeding" serves to degrade accuracy and coordination which results in disfluenices. Like going down stairs, if you choose to run down the flight of stairs you greatly increase the likelihood that you will trip and fall. If you proceed very slowly, placing each foot on each step and holding onto the railings with both hands, you will make it without falling, but it will take you a very long time to descend. There is a rate at which we can go down stairs both quickly and safely. That is the rate we seek for our client's speech; quick enough so it does not draw unfavorable attention to the speaker, but slow enough to minimize disfluencies.

Description

For most who stutter, slowing the speaking rate usually facilitates increased fluency. For some clients, it may afford them slightly more processing time when speaking: more time to find the appropriate words, more time to construct sentences, or more time to focus on the motor aspects of speaking. For still others, it may help combat feelings of being rushed to talk or other symptoms of anxiety. Regardless of the reason, speaking slowly has a very beneficial and profound effect on fluency.

How slow is slow enough? In general, the client needs to demonstrate that he is deliberately controlling the rate of his speech and the rate is markedly slower than his habitual rate. Most clients complain that slow speech sounds unnatural. Some even feel that slow speech is less desirable than their stuttering! In part, their perception of this speaking rate is distorted by their speaking anxieties and by the difference it creates in their speech. This difference is commonly discerned to be negative, even though speech is more fluent. Clients are often so sensitive about their speech, that any change, even a change that creates greater fluency, is difficult to adjust to. Others feel that their slow speech does not adequately reflect their mood or their personality. This is a legitimate complaint. Clients sometimes need to be urged to put these reservations aside temporarily and redirected to focus on speaking in a slower, controlled, and more fluent manner. A key component to the slow rate target is becoming disciplined as a speaker. This likely will be a different concept to the client as speaking is usually considered to be an automatic process; we are now requesting that speaking become a disciplined, deliberate activity and that the speaker take active control of the process. Although clients frequently complain that this is "extra work" for them to talk, the benefits are multifold and hard to deny.

Like learning any new skill, a slow rate requires the client to exaggerate the desired response, speaking so slowly that it is almost uncomfortable. As the client becomes more proficient he is allowed to increase his rate a little at a time, as long as his speech remains fluent. The idea is still not to speak automatically, but in a controlled fashion. The client's attention is also directed to sensing the motion of his articulators as he speaks, feeling the relaxed, almost effortless movements progressing from sound to sound as he articulates each word.

Slow rate activities usually begin by reading selected passages. Intensive feedback is a key ingredient in achieving the desired rate. Provide either corrective or positive feedback at least every 30 seconds for the first 3 minutes of an activity or until the client demonstrates the appropriate control. Reading enables the client to focus more on implementing the slow rate target as it does not require the client to generate his own ideas or formulate his own thoughts.

A reading activity can transition to become a conversational activity by asking the client's opinion on what he has just read. Clients commonly discontinue the slow rate target as soon as they are done with the activity, so you may need to re-instruct the client to continue to use slow rate as he moves into the conversation. Other activities might include a monologue (a 2- to 3-minute speech about a specific topic), making phone calls, introducing himself to new people, or giving an informational presentation. During activities that involve novel listeners, gestural cuing might be utilized for feedback so as not to detract from the client's speech or draw attention to it being a therapeutic activity. In all slow rate activities, draw the client's attention to the smooth, fluid and effortless movement from sound to sound as he speaks.

How is the client's performance measured? The most accurate way to measure speech rate is by counting words or syllables uttered per minute. However, the time required to calculate rate in this manner is untenable as the calculations take too long to be useful. A more functional measure is needed. The clinician begins by modeling a rate for the client to emulate and then provides intensive feedback based on the client's productions. The clinician must fix the model rate in memory to guide the client and judge his productions against.

Clients usually need a reason, in addition to improving fluency, to encourage them to use slow rate. Analogies or related life situations may be helpful to convince the client of the merits of using this target. There are a couple approaches that may be effective. The first is that of being a good communicator. It is the responsibility of an effective communicator to convey information to the listener. This is more than just "dumping" information (as quickly as possible) upon the listener; it entails insuring that the listener understands what the speaker has said. This can be facilitated by speaking at a slow rate, thus giving the listener time to process the information presented. If you have ever had a teacher in class who talks so rapidly that it takes all of your energy just to take notes, you understand this concept. An effective communicator speaks at a rate that enables the listener to think about, consider, and compare the new information with information they may already have. A teacher speaking slowly allows students to take notes and think about the ideas he or she is trying to convey. For the client to be a good communicator, it is necessary that he speak at a rate that enables the listener to not only hear, but also consider and understand what has been said.

Another approach focuses on the perceptions of confidence and authority of quick versus slower speakers. Individuals, such as corporate leaders, the Pope, and the President command respect and are viewed as "important," in part by their speech patterns. Their message is important enough that they speak it in a slow, relaxed, and deliberate style. The speech pattern of individuals perceived to have less credibility, say people trying to sell you something, are often typified by a rapid, unrelenting rate, so as not to give the listener time to think or disagree. Most clients who stutter already sensitive to the perceptions of others based on their speech, will respond to this example. Nonetheless, slow rate can be a very hard sell.

Instructions to the Client

Begin by explaining the purpose of this target: to take advantage of the fluency enhancing effects and to learn to be a disciplined speaker. Some who stutter may have speech motor systems that function better at a slower rate of speed and it's important to take advantage of this simple strategy. Once mastered, the client can then elect to utilize it in situations in which he feels the need. But mastering it requires that it be practiced intensively. Most clients will use this target in structured activities, but revert back to their old, habitual speaking pattern the very second the activity ends. This generally is because they haven't allowed themselves to be comfortable speaking in this manner because they feel that people will think their slow speech is peculiar, in spite of the fluency which emerges. Clinicians need to be very persistent in directing the client to use a slow rate.

> **Clinical Insight:** The clinician is often called on to provide reasons the client will find compelling to convince him to speak at this slow rate. One such rationale may be garnered from advice given to public speakers. People who stutter are often concerned about how others perceive their speech and therefore are interested in being thought of as a good communicator. Being a good communicator entails more than orally conveying information to an audience. Apart from being knowledgeable about the topic and organizing the information in a logical way, good communicators also need to take responsibility for audience members understanding what is being said. Although most focus almost exclusively on the encoding segment of the message, the decoding component of communication is equally or even more important. The speaker needs to present information in a way so that the listener will understand it. The instructor who talks so quickly that it requires all of your efforts just to write the notes is actually communicating pretty poorly. The instructor might be advised just to hand out his notes, because audience members focus so much energy on writing, they have few resources to think about what the words mean. The teacher is focusing on getting the quantity of information out, but not considering the quality of how it is being received. Good communicators speak at a rate which enables listeners to think about, analyze, and even ponder questions about the topic. A slower speaking rate enables that.
>
> Good children's storytellers don't read a book as fast as they can. They read slowly with inflection and intonation so that the children can build mental images of the story in the head. Slow rate is a prime feature of effective communication.

Remember that their habitual (quicker) rate is driven by anxiety. Two things happen when anxious; new behaviors are more difficult to learn and perception is skewed, meaning that the client's speech effectively isn't really as slow as the client perceives it to be. The clinician might say to the client, "*Most clients find this hard to do at first. The hardest time to change a behavior is when you are anxious. It seems under the pressures of being nervous that doing what you usually do is the easier route to take and most seem to do so without even thinking about it, even when you don't like the result (stuttering). That means that we will need to re-double our efforts and really focus on managing your rate. I will signal you when I first notice your rate speeding up, even just a little bit. Try to make the adjustment right away and maintain it for as long as you can. I will instruct you to stop speaking if it becomes too difficult for you. I think you will see that speaking slowly will be a valuable tool in diminishing your stuttering.*

That will help you feel less anxious about stuttering. Perhaps we'll record you reading the paragraph so we can listen together so you can hear how it sounds to others."

Slow speech takes some salesmanship. As previously mentioned, clients may respond better to use slow rate, thinking that it enhances their effectiveness as a communicator, which it generally does. People who stutter are commonly perceived to be nervous when they speak. Slowing the rate of speech goes a long way toward overcoming these perceptions.

It is important for the clinician to model the speaking rate that is desired from the client when describing the activity and the desired response from the client. This is usually the most effective teaching tool. The initial attempts at slow rate should be greatly exaggerated—How slow? Until it hurts! By beginning in a very exaggerated fashion, you will be able to ease up a bit and soon accept a slightly quicker rate. The critical element is that the client is controlling his speech, being disciplined, and speaking in a volitional manner. Slow rate can take some of the automaticity of speech away and some clients also diminish variations in intensity and intonation in the process. This often makes client feel like they sound like a robot. Explain that this is a natural reaction to first using the technique and it will change as he becomes more adept at using it.

The importance of learning to speech in a volitional, controlled manner cannot be overemphasized. It may be useful to have the client watch or listen to a recording of his slow rate. In most cases the recording helps the client come to the realization that their speech doesn't sound as exaggerated as they previously perceived it to be.

Suggested Materials

Reading aloud is usually a good speaking modality to start with because it enables the client to focus more of his attention on maintaining the slow rate. Additional effort is not expended on generating things to say. Have the client read a children's storybook as if he were reading it to a young child. Explain that the idea is not to demonstrate his speed-reading skills, but to allow the child the time necessary to envision what is happening in the story. This requires the reader to go slowly and even use inflections and intonation too.

Conversation is the most common mode of speaking. You may wish the client to read a brief paragraph, and then explain what he has just read or offer his opinion about the topic. Ideally, he will continue to use a slow speaking rate in the transition from reading to conversation; but it is not uncommon for a client to need frequent cuing to do so at first.

You could also prepare a PowerPoint presentation with pictures of local landmarks. Have the client talk about these points of interest using his slow rate. Comment on how his slower rate can make the presentation more interesting to the listeners and gives them time to think about the information he is communicating, and maybe formulate some questions about it. Using a slow rate is like giving a performance almost as another character. If fact, having the client emulate someone with a slow speaking rate (like Mr. Rogers) is another means of getting him to use the slow rate target.

Using a slow rate brings up another irony of stuttering. For clients who want so badly not to stutter, using this easy and very effective target often seems like too great a sacrifice to make!

Voice Onset

Client Profile

A characteristic of Maria's stuttering is an abrupt voice onset. Subconsciously trying to overcome the possibility that she will stutter at the beginning of a sentence, Maria uses extra effort to begin each utterance. Perhaps she thinks that by using more muscular force as she begins speaking that she can overpower the stuttering block. Watching her closely, it can be noted that she takes a rather deep, quick inhalation of air just before starting a sentence. This is much more than is normally required; it's almost as if she was going to shout to someone across the room. The usual result of this is for her speech to start with a "jerk," almost like when you try to talk while lifting something heavy. It's very noticeable to everyone and they often see that something's wrong with the way she speaks right away.

Rationale

One of the parts of speaking that perhaps requires the most coordination is the precise moment when voicing is initiated. Laryngeal blocks result from excessive muscular effort used to adduct the vocal folds in the process of phonating. This usually occurs when the speaker is anxious or worries about being unable to start the utterance. Most people who stutter seem to have a natural tendency to speak more forcefully under these conditions. Their fear serves to tense the vocal folds prematurely and the speaker feels the need to push harder to start phonation. These fears usually increase after a series of unsuccessful attempts, resulting in a habit pattern that can be difficult to change.

Most people who stutter do not stutter when they whisper. Whispering differs from speaking in only one aspect, the element of voicing. By reducing the complexity of the speaking process, fluency will more likely be the result. When difficulty with voice onset is a component of the client's disfluency, working to ease the muscular effort used to vocalize may benefit the client. Recalling that speaking is a very complex, highly integrated process that simplifying the process should result in greater fluency is actually quite logical.

Speaking to the patient, the clinician might explain, "*The very beginning of an utterance is the most critical point of speaking; it's also the most complicated part in terms of movement as well. In an instant we change our respiration pattern from resting to breathing for speech. We have an idea and need to scan our brain for the right words to express out thought and the grammar to string the words together properly. We formulate a motor program to articulate all the sounds strung together in the sentence as well and the intonation and inflection patterns to give it subtle meanings. We bring our vocal folds together to make voice and begin to move the structures in our mouth with a high degree of precision to correctly make the sounds. Research has shown us that formulating and beginning the motor program for speaking takes more brain activity for people who stutter. Like many things, if we slow down the process and go a little easier, there often is a better result. I want you to focus your attention on relaxing your throat and bringing your vocal folds together very gently to begin producing your voice. Try it with me."*

Phonation begins when the vocal folds come together as we begin to exhale. When more effort than necessary is used to adduct the vocal folds, the folds are not free to vibrate and a block results. The Vocal Onset technique focuses the client's attention on managing the muscular effort utilized to adduct the vocal folds when beginning to exhale. This technique ensures that the vocal folds begin in an abducted position (apart) by allowing a little more exhalated air than usual to escape just prior to bringing the vocal folds together for phonation. Phonation is initiated by moving the vocal folds together in a slow, gentle manner, avoiding the excessive tension that causes blocking.

Description

Some people who stutter exhibit laryngeal blocks in which the vocal folds are adducted so tightly that exhaled air cannot escape or it escapes in sudden, uncontrolled bursts. These blocks prohibit phonation, and thereby interfere significantly with speech fluency. To address laryngeal blocks, the vocal onset target is utilized to ensure that the vocal folds do not "lock" in adducted position, and that airflow is not obstructed so that vocalization can begin in a smooth, easy manner.

The vocal onset technique slows down and slightly modifies the normal process of producing voice. This modification affects the timing and effort in bringing the vocal folds together for phonation. Normally, just as inhalation changes to exhalation, the vocal folds are approximated and then begin to vibrate as air flows between them. Using minimal muscular effort to adduct the vocal folds at the moment of voice onset allows more air to escape as the vocal folds are begin brought together. Figure 3–3 shows the normal cycle of respiration for speech, comprised of a rapid inhalation of air, followed by an extended exhalation. Note that the vocal folds are brought together for phonation very soon after the point at which the speaker begins the exhalation process. By delaying slightly the point at which the vocal folds are adducted, more air escapes before phonate begins (Figure 3–4). If exaggerated, an audible /h/ sound can be heard, indicating that the airway is not obstructed. When demonstrating that the airway is unobstructed, the client begins a slow, gradual, easy movement to bring his vocal folds together to produce voice. Vocal intensity is gradually allowed to rise and the client then begins to articulate the word, moving from the first vocalized sound to the next subsequent sound. The overall effect is like slowly sliding into the word. This is done on the first word of each utterance.

The client is instructed, *"You often have difficulty initiating an utterance because your airway is blocked by your vocal folds closing too tightly. As a result, your breathing is obstructed and therefore you cannot produce a voice. To overcome that tendency, I would like you to begin*

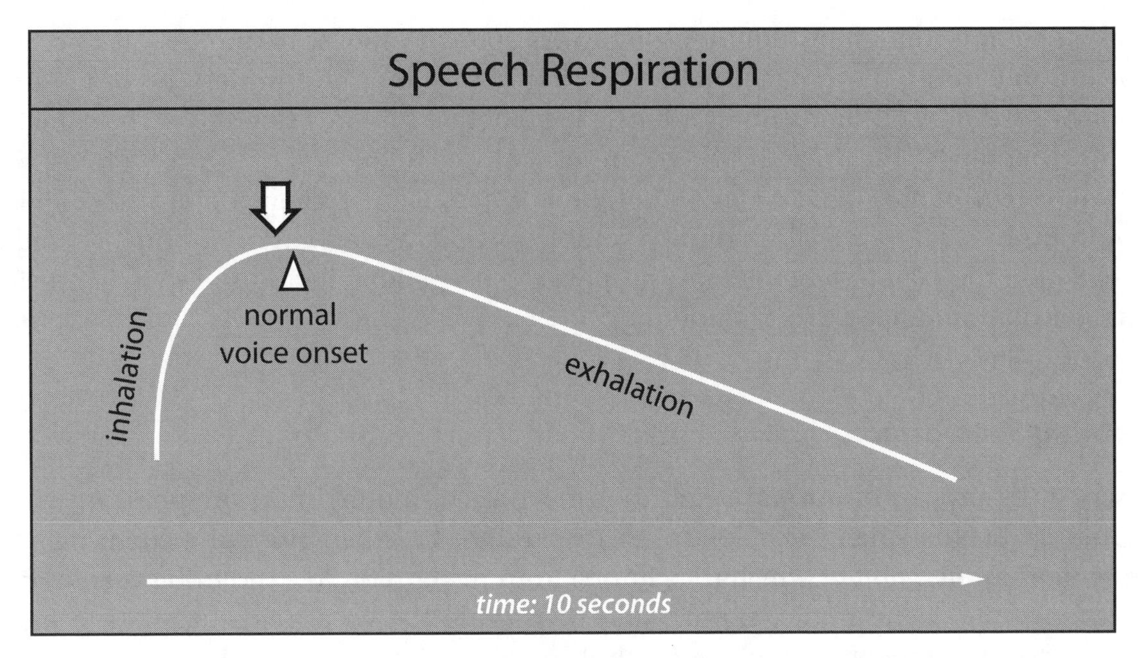

Figure 3–3. Respiration for speech.

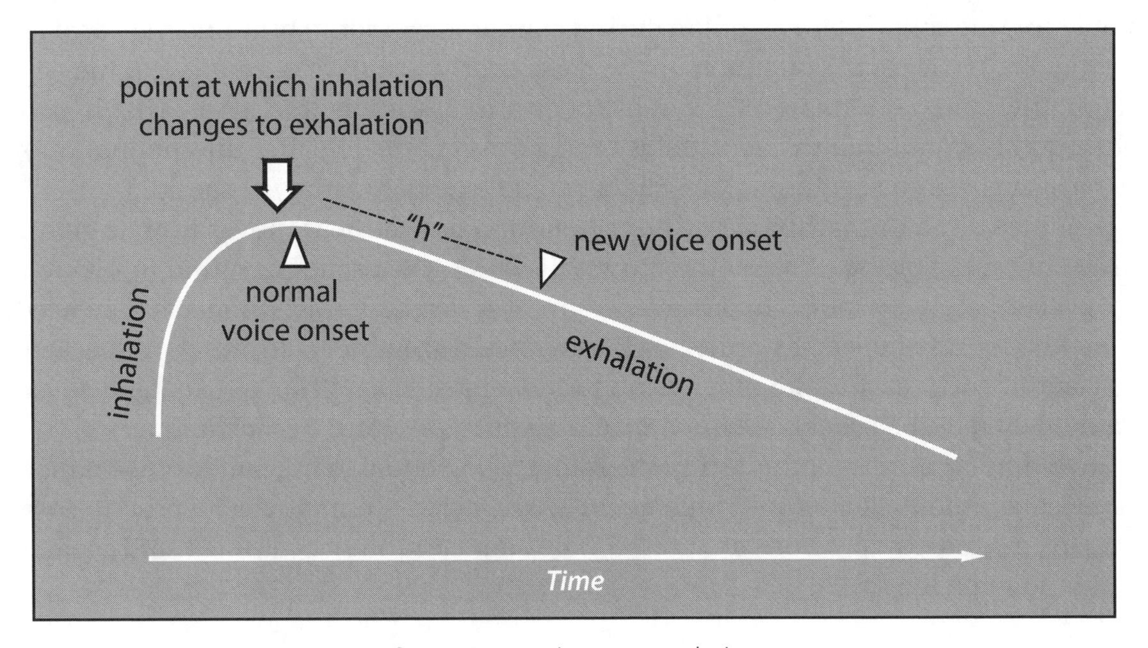

Figure 3–4. Voice onset technique

each utterance by letting some air escape before you bring your vocal folds together to make your voice. Acoustically it sounds like you are making an /h/ sound at the beginning of words. After you hear the /h/ sound, bring your vocal folds together gently and begin voicing the first sound. Let's start by practicing saying these words aloud. Remember, start each word with the /h/ sound."

At first it is desirable to exaggerate the duration of the onset of phonation to ensure that the production is in the client's volitional control. Clients usually try to speed up the process, but it is important that they remain disciplined when speaking. As they become more adept at using the target, usually after several sessions, the duration can be reduced, as long as the client demonstrates that he can smoothly initiate phonation. The clinician listens carefully for the /h/ sound to ensure the delayed adduction of the vocal folds.

The intent of the vocal onset technique is to reduce the client's fear of becoming caught up in a laryngeal block and be unable to work loose. Mastery of this technique should give the client more confidence speaking, thereby reducing the muscle tension that contributes to instances of stuttering.

Teaching Suggestions

Describe the process of normal respiration for speech, highlighting the point at which phonation begins when the vocal folds are brought together. Have the client demonstrate, noting the point at which the change from inspiration to exhalation takes place. Next, have the client inhale, exhale, and then bring the vocal folds together to make voice. Instruct the client to inhale and exhale a second time, but delay bringing the vocal folds together by about two seconds before starting to phonate. The vocal folds should be approximated very softly, using a minimum of muscular effort. There must be an audible /h/ (the sound of air escaping during exhalation) prior to bringing the vocal folds together. Focus the client's attention on the easy, effortless start of phonation at the beginning of utterances. It is this *feeling* that is important for the client to learn. The /h/ sound is the audible signal that the vocal folds have not yet come together and phonation has not yet started. In the beginning, the client should exaggerate the /h/ sound.

Begin teaching this technique by just phonating as the client moves from inhalation to exhalation to voicing. Proceed then to single words, then sentences, and finally to use in conversation. In sentences and conversation, the vocal onset technique is only needed on the first sound of the first word of each utterance. Take time to ensure that the client is proficient at each level before progressing to the next speaking mode. Exaggerated clinician modeling and feedback are important aspects in teaching this technique.

The primary purpose of this technique is to develop a tool to prevent laryngeal blocks. The most common client errors using vocal onset include failing to allow the release of sufficient exhalated air before phonating, not adducting the vocal folds softly enough, and trying to go too fast.

Suggested Materials

Prepare a list of words beginning with the /h/ sound. Since the vocal onset technique utilizes the /h/ sound to insure that air is escaping, /h/-initial words can serve a dual purpose when first learning this technique. Words beginning with plosive sounds are not appropriate for the voice onset technique because they require a complete closure of the vocal folds, obstructing of the exhalated air. This is the opposite of the way the voice onset technique works.

- Using the same word list, have the client generate sentences beginning with words starting with the /h/ sound. There are also several prepared passages available which contain a high proportion of /h/ words.
- Bring a collection of pictures into the session and have the client ask *wh*-questions (using the voice onset technique) about the pictures.

Light Articulatory Contacts

Case Profile

Doug's stuttering sounds as though he is struggling to make each sound; it seems very labored and he appears to use extra muscular effort in articulating some sounds. It looks like he is forcing his mouth to move to form many of the sounds. His effortful speech attracts a great deal of attention from his listeners. It lacks the smooth, easy transitions from sound to sound, almost like walking wearing concrete boots. Doug is very aware that words that begin with /b/, /p/, /w/, /k/, and /g/ are more difficult for him to say. Sometimes, he even substitutes another word for one he knows will be troublesome. When stuttering, it looks like Doug is working very hard to speak and others feel sorry for him because of his labored speech movements.

Rationale

Repetitions, prolongations, or blocks are often the associated with utilizing too much muscular effort when articulating sounds. Basically, sounds are made by moving the structures within the oral cavity; the production of some sounds is a function of structures coming into contact with one another. For example, the /p/ is made by bringing the upper and lower lips into contact momentarily, and then releasing the contact as air pressure builds within the oral cavity. The bilabial contact only needs to be enough to let the intraoral air pressure rise slightly. Only a minimal amount of muscular effort is required to do this. Some stuttering is the result of using more effort than is necessary to make the contact, sort of "muscling" or "overpowering" it. When this happens, the smooth flow of speech is interrupted.

Many who stutter have learned (or believe) that some sounds are more difficult for them to say. To compensate for their predicted difficulty, they often use more muscular force articulating feared sounds than is necessary. Light Articulatory Contacts focus the client's attention on using minimal and appropriate muscular effort for speech. They learn to monitor their proprioceptive feedback while speaking to ensure that their oral musculature is relaxed when articulating sounds and speaking.

Description

When most sounds are formed during the articulatory process, aspects of the tongue, palate, lips and teeth come into contact with other oral structures to modify or restrict the outward flow of exhaled air. In most instances, only a minimal amount of muscular effort is necessary to bring these articulators into contact with one another to produce the desired physical and acoustic effect. The pressure required at the point of contact is quite minimal. But, if too much effort is used, the articulatory contacts are slowed or otherwise impaired. For people who stutter, this excessive effort can result in blocks, repetitions, or prolongations of sounds. The normal effortless motion of speaking is changed in a way somewhat analogous to stomping your feet when you walk. The extra effort is not needed, and serves only to slow your overall speed and interfere with the precision of your movements.

To compensate for the tendency to articulate in this forcible manner, the client is asked to monitor his or her articulatory contacts so as to control each contact using minimal force, much like tip-toeing while walking. By attending to these proprioceptive motor aspects of speaking, the speaker reduces the likelihood that disfluencies will occur. Some sounds are not produced by making contact, such as the vowels sounds and sounds like the phoneme /r/. Light articulatory contacts usually are not effective in addressing these specific sounds.

Instructions to Client

Review the anatomy and physiology of speaking from the first session. Highlight some of the anatomic and physiologic aspects of normal articulation for the client. Use a mirror so the client can see, hear, and feel how certain sounds are produced. Begin with more "visible" sounds, such as /p/, /f/, or /t/. Ask the client to note which structures make contact to produce each of these sounds.

Next, have the client make the /p/ in a very easy, effortless manner; then contrast that production with one using much more muscular effort. Usually, the client will identify the effortful production attempt as feeling more like stuttering. Have the client make other "easy-hard" contrasts, especially with the sounds that he or she reports as being difficult or on which he frequently stutters. Label the "easy" production as an example of a "light contact" and have the client read a list of words beginning with that sound, practicing the light contact technique. With success, move to sentences and then to conversation, using light contacts on specific sounds.

Using light contacts and minimal muscular effort to articulate sounds usually enhances fluency overall by minimizing blocks, repetitions, and prolongations. This speaking pattern is often in sharp contrast to what the client has learned to do, and therefore will require more monitoring and concentration than is usual.

Sometimes, in describing the extra effort used in speaking, the client is asked to place his hand, palm down on the table. To demonstrate an effortful (hard) articulatory

Clinician Tip: The key to light articulatory contacts comes in developing the speaker's awareness of the proprioceptive feedback while speaking (the feeling of speech). This becomes another tool in monitoring the muscular effort for speaking and listening for disfluencies. The client needs to be aware when too much effort is being used in articulating sounds and accept the responsibility for making appropriate adjustments when it becomes too effortful.

contact, press your hand firmly down on top of the client's to represent the effort used in articulating the sound. To contrast it and demonstrate a light articulatory contact, touch the top of the client's hand very softly, reflecting the effort used in this manner of production. This paints a visual, acoustic, and tactile picture contrasting hard and light contacts during the articulatory process.

During structured speaking activities using light contacts, periodically ask the client to report the amount of effort he is using in articulating feared sounds. This process of frequently monitoring his own effort articulating is part of what we want the client to learn to do for himself. When used immediately in advance of making feared sounds, light articulatory contacts are used to avoid having disfluencies. However, it is valuable practice to use light articulatory contacts on all sounds to get the feel of taking responsibility and controlling speaking.

Often, the sounds that a client finds difficult to say are those in his own name. Instruct the client to watch him- or herself in the mirror saying his or her name when at home alone. Have the client feel the muscle movements and physical contact saying his or her name while driving in the car. Speaking is largely a motor skill and practicing in nonthreatening environments can also be very valuable.

Suggested Materials

- Prepare lists of single words beginning with the sound(s) the client fears or that you have noted that he has difficulty with.
- Construct sentences from these words in various positions within the sentence.
- Use the list of single words to have the client utilize each word in a sentence he must generate.
- Have the client read the word list to a person unfamiliar to him.
- Provide a list of restaurants for the client to call and make a dinner reservation in his name. Call back the next day to cancel it.
- Talk with an unknown person, working feared words into the conversation as frequently as possible.

Syllable Stretch

Client Profile

Charlie seems to speak pretty rapidly and as a consequence, it is hard for him to use any target; his anxiety overwhelms the effective control of his speech. Fluency enhancing targets require the speaker to be very disciplined while talking, and Charlie struggles with that. His nervousness makes it hard for him to speak in a different manner; he always seems to fall back to what he usually does, which leads to more stuttering. Sometimes, he is aware that he is out of control, but can't seem to slow himself down so he can use his targets. He sounds as though he is speeding to get his words out before he stutters again. As a result he sounds like he's racing from one stuttering block to the next.

Rationale

To the extent that fluency improves as the motor movements of speech are slowed down and brought into the speaker's intentional control, syllable stretch can be an effective training exercise. From a different perspective, we see that people who stutter do not stutter when they sing. One of the differences between singing and speaking is that the vowel sounds are lengthened in song. Some have pointed to making the transition between sounds as a source of difficulty for those who stutter. The syllable stretch technique encompasses both of these phenomenon; slowing the rate of movement during speech and stretching the vowels sounds in the words.

Speaking in this manner requires a good deal of discipline on the part of the speaker. Like all fluency enhancing targets, syllable stretching is based in normal speech production, but the resulting sound of the speech is by definition distorted. This is troublesome for some clients. The therapeutic intent of this technique is to help the client develop discipline as a speaker and build a motoric model of speech which flows from one sound to the next.

Description

A well-disciplined syllable stretch entails holding each vowel sound for two seconds while articulating each word. This is done in a manner that stretches words and links them together, preserving the continuous character of speech production.

Clinical Insight: Don't be surprised if your client's initial reaction to syllable stretching is not immediately positive. People who stutter are often very sensitive to how their speech sounds, and syllable stretching usually sounds different to them, and not in a good way. Therapy is about becoming a more disciplined speaker and learning to speak in different ways which lead to controlled fluency. But clients often feel that speaking in this manner sounds robotic or they fear people will think they sound intoxicated with slurred speech. Encourage your client to look beyond this initial reaction and recognize the longer term benefit. By analogy, walking on a treadmill can be thought of as somewhat ridiculous—walking is a means of getting from one point to another. But walking on a treadmill takes you nowhere! However, the overall goal is not to walk and go nowhere, it's to build cardiofitness or lose weight. Standing in one place and walking can seem a bit ridiculous, but the longer term benefits may be worth the effort.

Instructions to the Client

The clinician might anticipate a degree of resistance from the patient when introducing the syllable stretch target. A firm, yet encouraging attitude will help sell this technique to the client. Clients should be willing to try it in the clinic if they feel safe experimenting with their speech. However, the client's willingness to try it in other locations might not be as great.

The clinician might introduce syllable stretch as follows; *"Using any target requires a pretty high degree of discipline and I'd like to try a new target today that will require you to think a lot about using it. I'm going to ask you to stretch the vowel sound in each syllable of the words you speak for two full seconds. The speech will sound a little different, and some don't like how it sounds, but there are two things that I'd like you to learn for using syllable stretch. First, that becoming a more disciplined speaker will benefit your fluency and it is a key element to your future success. Second, I want you to feel your muscle movements as you transition from sound to sound. If you pay less attention to the sound of your speech you will be better able to focus on the muscle movements as you move effortlessly from sound to sound.*

"Let me demonstrate what I'd like you to do. I'm going to say the word 'alphabet' stretching out the vowel sounds for two seconds each. Listen carefully, 'aaaaaaaaalphaaaaaaaaabeeeeeeeet.' I'm going to ask you to say the word the exact same way and feel how easy and relaxed your muscle movement becomes. Are you ready? Give it a try."

The clinician should ask the client to reflect on his or her production. It may also be prudent to acknowledge that speaking in the manner sounds different than regular speech. This may appease the client's need to object to the sound of his utterance, at least temporarily, and stay focused on being a disciplined speaker and the feel of moving smoothly from one sound to the next.

Suggested Materials

Most clients begin at the word level, so the clinician should prepare a list of single words. Starting out with words that begin with a vowel sound may be preferable as the client begins by stretching the first sound he encounters. Guide the client to a full 2-second stretch by giving him feedback and encouraging him to exaggerate the stretch.

After some practice, the next step might be short (three-word) sentences. Make sure that a full 2 seconds is used in stretching. The client can progress to longer sentences, monologues and conversations as his performance level allows. Again, focus the client's attention to the feel of the muscle movements while speaking and speaking in a disciplined manner.

Continuous Phonation

Client Profile

The speech motor skills Jim demonstrates in his speech appear to be poorly coordinated; sometimes there is a degree of imprecision and even slurring when he articulates. A few sound productions are slightly distorted and he occasionally mispronounces words every now and then. Jim's stuttering improves when he speaks at a slower rate or when he whispers. His speech sounds a bit labored and he seems to be working very hard to talk.

Rationale

Some clients appear to have more difficulty than others with the motor aspects of speaking, particularly when anxious. It often happens that making the act of speaking less complex for clients and improves their performance and fluency. Slow rate is one example of making speaking less complex; whispering is another.

Speaking slower requires less skill and tends not to test the speaker's abilities. Imagine a job packing tiny, delicate glass vases into a box that holds 12 vases. The employee needs to carefully pick up one vase at a time and gently place it into the box without breaking the vase or any other vases. Most people would be capable of a high level of success at this task, if they could take their time. But what if you were required to fill the box in less than 15 seconds? The likelihood of breaking the merchandise is inversely proportional to the time allotted to do the task. That is to say, breakage increases as time decreases. The same holds true for speaking. Say the phrase "toy boat." Say it 10 times. Finally, say it 10 times in 4 seconds. As your speed increases, you accuracy decreases. For the client who stutters, simplifying speaking improves performance. Reducing rate increases fluency.

From phonetics we learn that some of the sounds in our language are voiced and some are unvoiced. When we speak, our voice is constantly being "turned on and off" to correctly articulate the sounds we speak. But if we simplify speech by speaking without voicing (whispering), people who stutter generally experience more fluency. The same holds true for leaving our voice on all the time, continuously phonating while we speak. This is the basis of the continuous phonation technique.

Furthermore, we observe that, in singing, there is a much greater voicing component when utterances are sung. We see that people who stutter don't stutter when they sing. Continuous voicing (phonation) takes advantage of these factors to facilitate fluency.

Description

Continuous phonation sounds a little like the chanting of monks in a monastery or cathedral. It also sounds a little like singing, except the range is not as great. Like chanting, there is a degree of vocal inflection and intonation that overlays the utterance. For continuous phonation, the component of voicing is intentionally "on" as much as possible. It does not matter that voiceless sounds become voiced ("came" becomes "game," its voiced cognate). The overall effect is a smooth, effortless, and melodious speech production.

> **Clinical Insight:** Some clients tend not to what to think about speaking and believe if they can take their mind off of their speech that it will be fluent. It is only when they "overthink" and worry about their speech that bad things happen. This line of thought leaves their fluency up to fate or luck. Unfortunately, when the pressure is on, their luck usually comes up short and they stutter. A basic premise of stuttering therapy is for the client to take responsibility for speaking fluently. Therapy gives him the tools to do so. Clients must feel empowered to change their stuttering; they need to know that there is something that they can do to manage fluent speech. Stuttering isn't the client's fault, but it is his or her responsibility to be fluent.

Instructions to the Client

Clients should be instructed in determining whether they are voicing or not. Their attention can be drawn to the thyroid cartilage to feel when there is vibration and their voice is on. At first, have the client repeat a word over and over, maintaining voicing throughout.

Words beginning with the /m/ sound may be a good choice as the client begins by voicing the first sound of the word. The clinician demonstrates, "*Mine, mine, mine, mine, mine, mine,*" keeping her voice on continuously throughout her utterance. The client echoes her words.

Next the clinician models a sentence, voicing all of the words in the chantlike manner. "*Mine is the red coat on the right.*" "*Maybe you could look in the other room?*" The client mimics her speech and receives feedback on his attempt from the clinician.

The clinician might explain this target to the client like this; "*We're going to try a new target which simplifies speaking a bit. It's sort of like singing, but more like chanting; have you ever heard a chant? What I will ask you to do is to use your voice all of the time when you speak. Normally, we turn our voice on and off as some sounds, like /m/, are voiced and some, like /p/ are unvoiced. So to simplify speech, we will voice all the sounds. It sounds like this; 'My dog likes to walk in the park with me everyday morning.' Did you hear that my voice was on throughout the entire utterance? You try to do the same thing.*

"*You can feel your throat to tell whether you are using your voice all of the time. You did very well, and I want to try some more. Did you feel how smooth and easy your speech became? Eventually we will work to make your speech that smooth, but without needing to use continuous phonation, but for now I think we will want to practice it some more. Let's have a conversation and both use it.*"

Clients generally are reluctant to use continuous phonation in public. Its value is in speaking in a different way, which is more conducive to fluency and does not deal directly with stuttering. It should promote the client's awareness of speaking more slowly and in a disciplined manner. Being controlled and speaking in a manner that enhances fluency is the lesson learned from continuous phonation.

Suggested Materials

Have a list of words beginning with the /m/ sound. Prepare a list of sentences that have words beginning with /m/ embedded in them. Clients generally work their way up to the conversational level fairly rapidly. Begin conversations with very neutral topics that won't stir the client's interest too much. Later, the client can be challenged by discussing topics that he feels more passionate about, perhaps a political candidate, a special interest, or a cause that he supports.

Stuttering Modification Targets

Learning to take control of moments of stuttering. The orientation of these therapy techniques shares the common feature of modifying the client's stuttering pattern and providing a means for the client to gain control of his stuttering. Although fluency-enhancing targets are modeled after the normal speaking process, stuttering modification targets give the client tools to work through and control the instances of stuttering that inevitably will occur. Most of the stuttering modifications techniques were developed by or are derivatives of the work of Van Riper (1996).

Pull-Out

Client Profile

Tim's blocks last for almost 15 seconds, but to him, it feels like an eternity. He feels like a victim of his stuttering because he is unable to free himself from his stuttering blocks. As he struggles through each block, people stare. This only makes Tim more self-conscious and embarrassed by them. Because he can't do anything to get past these disfluencies, he lives in constant fear of them happening the next time. Tim seems always tense and nervous about speaking. His attempts to get through each disfluency only seem to make his stuttering worse. He feels helpless to do anything about his situation.

Rationale

The anxiety that results from being afraid of stuttering increases tension in the muscles used to speak and produce voice. These fears are heightened by being unable to get out of stuttering blocks. Clients instinctively attempt to use more muscular force to fight their way out of the blocks, creating even greater struggle behaviors. It is curious that even though these attempts usually are ineffective in getting free from the stuttering, clients continue to use them over and over again, with the same result.

Pull-outs are a means of manipulating the stuttering block by gradually reducing, rather than increasing, muscular effort while blocking. The benefits are twofold. First, pull-outs allow the speaker to reduce struggle behaviors, which make his stuttering look less overtly severe to others. Second, pull-outs serve to break up the client's habit pattern, changing his stuttering behaviors. Changing the habituated patterns of stuttering enable the speaker to gain some control over his stuttering and thereby feel less anxious about speaking and less fearful of stuttering. This serves to reduce his overall muscle tension which promotes greater natural fluency.

Description

When the client is in the middle of a stuttering block, he learns to ease the amount of muscular effort, instead of escalating it. In effect, he "let's the block go," slipping out of it instead of using more force, trying "to muscle through it" or overpower it.

Habits can be hard to break, especially habits that are formed due to fear. Learning a new behavior while in a fearful or anxious state is challenging. However, pull-outs are tools that empower clients to control their stuttering and the reward, therefore, is great. Pulling out of a block gives the sensation of stretching it until it becomes malleable. There are stages in the process of employing the pull-out. First the client needs to recognize he or she is having a block. Although this may seem obvious to those who don't stutter, think of it as though you are slipping and falling while walking tensely on an icy sidewalk. At a certain point, after you've slipped, you are aware of what's happening. But by the time you can put it into words. "Boom! You're on the ground." We are asking the client to recognize what is happening, then do something that is not his natural instinct to do. A second step for the client is to determine the site of the muscular tension and feel its force. Finally, the client is asked to slowly diminish this muscle tension and release from the block. Unlike the example of slipping and falling on the sidewalk, the client will have more time to dedicate to the task of modifying his stuttering block. However, the first attempts are usually awkward until the client gets the feel of being able to release from the block more gracefully and with less effort. Eventually, he or she can become skilled at this release and at that point it will be a valued tool in controlling stuttering.

Clinical Insight: The pull-out technique is very empowering for clients, giving them a first sense of actually being able to control something that seemed uncontrollable. For some, it is a turning point and motivator in their therapy. At last there is something within their power to do about stuttering moments. Using pull-outs, initially the process of easing out of a stutter can take a while and it seems the stutter and the client are each battling for control. With practice, however, clients can become skilled at modifying blocks. At this point, they have less to be fearful of "*If I stutter, I won't be stuck; I can use a pull-out and get out of it*!" With less fear, there is less muscle tension and fewer blocks and disfluency result.

It is somewhat ironic that clients continue to respond to their blocks in the same way, time after time, even though it isn't effective. In doing so, their stuttering becomes stronger and stronger, and the feelings that there is nothing that can be done about it grow. Therefore, the clinician serves as the agent of change; the coach who provides the insight that the client cannot see. This is the insight that leads to a successful change; one that empowers the client.

Instructions to the Client

Explain what is happening when the client experiences a stuttering block and how he typically responds to it, trying to force his way through it. Describe the block in terms of its location and the muscles that are involved. Share the observation that the client gives the appearance of fighting each block by using more muscular force in attempting to overcome it. This is a natural reaction to getting stuck. But, the more force he uses, the more struggle that results. The situation is somewhat analogous to Chinese finger traps or Finger Cuffs. One's natural instinct is to pull your fingers out, but the harder you try to pull your fingers from the cuff, the harder it is to escape. You need to go against your instincts and push your fingers together to release yourself from the trap. With stuttering, there is the same instinct, to push your way through. However, the client needs to learn to "stutter smarter," instead of yielding to his instincts.

It is sometimes easier to have the client imitate a stuttering block when first learning this technique because the stuttering block won't be as intense and it will start out under the client's control. Therefore, altering it will be easier. Have the client block and direct his attention to the focus of the disfluency; instruct him to feel the muscular pressure at the site of the block. Next, ask the client to gradually release the tension of the block and stretch into the next sound, continuing the word. It is often helpful to have the client watch himself in a mirror to better understand what is happening. Afterward, discuss the process of having a block and gradually working out of it by releasing the muscle tension, moving on with the rest of the sentence.

The clinician might explain it like this. *"I've noticed when you have a block that you try to force through it. That seems to result in more struggle behaviors and makes your stuttering look even more pronounced. What I'd like you to try instead, is to ease out of the block instead of fighting against it. Others have found this 'pull-out' technique easier to learn by faking a block, then easing out of it. First, have a block, then focus your attention on the where the muscle tension is. Next, gradually reduce the amount of tension and move along to the next sound in the word. Let me model it for you so you can see what I would like you to do."*

Suggested Materials

It is often beneficial to have the client watch himself in a mirror while he is learning pull-outs. This provides another sensory modality for feedback; now the client can watch, hear, and feel the pull-out. Of the three modalities, the feel of easing out of a block is the most important because it is the feel of moving through the block and the gradual release of muscular tension that will guide his efforts.

Clients often are more likely to stutter on specific sounds; usually sounds that they are very aware of and fear. After imitating disfluencies, you will be ready to guide the client through real stuttering blocks. Start out with a list of single words comprised of those the client feels are the most difficult to say. Continue to practice until the client demonstrates the ability to "feel his way" through his stuttering blocks. Reassure the client that, with practice, he will be able to manage blocks even easier and more efficiently. Move along to sentences and paragraphs before practicing the technique in conversation. Remember that each client moves at his own pace. Take the time necessary to master this target; this target will pay dividends by being able to rely on it when stuttering eventually returns. Having something to fall back on is always reassuring.

Bouncing

Client Profile

When Matt blocks he struggles so hard that his whole face turns red. His entire body freezes and yet, the harder he tries to speak, the worse his stuttering becomes. Matt has stuttered for quite a while. He's had therapy before in elementary school, but according to Matt, *"It didn't work 'cause I still stutter even worse than before."* His stuttering seems hopeless; he's read a lot about stuttering but just can't seem to change how he speaks. Matt's suffered through high school and is becoming worried about making new friends and needing to talk in classes when he is away at college next year. He even wonders what kind of job he will be able to get if he can't talk.

Rationale

Like pull-outs, bouncing is a means of breaking up a long-standing stuttering pattern. In learning to modify a behavior, any change is acceptable at first because is demonstrates that the client is able to do something differently. In time, however, the clinician seeks to reinforce those behavioral changes that approximate the desired speech outcome most closely. This is the principle of successive approximation. Unlike pull-outs, bouncing may be viewed more as an intermediate step toward controlling stuttering in that it generally serves a shorter term purpose.

There are two ways to use bouncing. Instead of pulling out of a stuttering block (the pull-out technique), the client may be encouraged to "bounce" out of it instead, another means of breaking up the muscular tension underlying the block. Bouncing works best when employed as a means of overcoming an anticipated block. For example, if the client typically stuttered on the word "baseball," he could begin the word by bouncing on it: "Ba - ba - ba - baseball." This is subtly different from a stuttering repetition in that the objective is to bounce using less muscular tension on each successive repetition of the syllable until the tension is normalized and the client can say the rest of the word in the appropriate, relaxed manner. The intent is to develop a means of controlling the stutter.

The second use for bouncing comes in stuttering on purpose, or having the client advertise his stuttering. Each of these intends to desensitize clients to their stuttering by reducing avoidances and letting listeners know that there may be further disfluencies in the client's speech. In this section, comments are directed to using bouncing for the first purpose, changing the client's habitual stuttering pattern.

Description

A client's belief that he will stutter on a specific sound or word can serve to cause his muscles to begin to tense in preparation to say the word. This attempt to say the sound or word typically is accompanied by more muscular effort than is necessary. As a result, stuttering occurs and the habitual struggle behaviors ensue. To break free from the hold of the block, the client repeats or bounces on the disfluent sound, reducing his muscular efforts as he continues bouncing along. Although bouncing can also be used to get free from a block, it is more effective if the client employs it just as he begins to utter the feared word. In this way, less tension builds up as bouncing serves to dissipate it before it has an opportunity to increase. In this way the client affects control over his stuttering moments.

Bouncing seems to work best on sounds in which the lips are used in its production, although many sounds can be bounced. By bouncing, the client learns another tool by which he may modify his stuttering pattern and gain control.

> **Clinical Insight:** Clients tend to like bouncing less than pull-outs because in their mind, bouncing is more akin to actual stuttering. However, the difference is that bouncing is an intention act, whereas stuttering is involuntary. Some see bouncing as a way of "playing with speech" likely in that there is less struggle involved in speaking. Others, however, may be less tolerant of any disfluencies in their speech and are miffed at why someone would want to stutter intentionally. But, being able to stutter in new and different ways remains an important step in breaking the habitual pattern.

Instructions to the Client

"We are going to try to stutter in different ways to help break up your habitual stuttering pattern that has developed over the years. I suggest that we start in a very simple way as undoing the pattern often is tricky work. What I will ask you to do is to repeat the first syllable of each word you expect to have trouble saying; that's called 'bouncing.' Make each successive bounce lighter and easier until you've reached a normal muscle tension level for fluent speech. We'll start by imitating a stuttering block so you can get the feel of bouncing on the first syllable, bouncing more gently with each syllable repetition. Let's start by reading these single words aloud, bouncing on the first syllable five or six times. Listen to me first. 'Wa-wa-wa-wa-wastebasket.' Now you try it. I want you to feel the muscle tension go away as you proceed."

Lead the client into reading sentences, and then have a conversation. In the beginning, you may wish the client to bounce on every word, just so he gets the feel of it. As he proceeds, the tension that is usually a part of his speech should diminish greatly. He is now stuttering in a different way; a much more volitional way. When stuttering becomes voluntary, it becomes easier to control.

Suggested Materials

Start with a list of single words beginning with plosive sounds (/p/ and /b/ for example) because they are very "visible" sounds in terms of how they are produced and they are commonly stuttered by most clients. Also compose a list of 20 sentences that incorporate words beginning with plosive sounds. Have a mirror available for the client to watch his productions. Conversation is another speaking mode for the client to try his bouncing speech. Conversations can be spontaneous or the clinician may wish to prepare a few topics to discuss.

Some clients dislike the bouncing technique because, to them, it is stuttering. However, the difference is that stuttering is involuntary and bouncing is done intentionally. If stuttering were to become all voluntary, then the client could elect not to stutter. But, for now, the focus is on stuttering in a different way; being able to break up the long-established patterned behaviors. Then the habit pattern can be changed in a way that minimizes stuttering. Remember, the desired outcome is controlled stuttering.

Voluntary Stutters

Client Profile

Shannon is hypersensitive to her disfluencies. She tends to overreact when she stutters and seems to find it very upsetting. She changes words a good deal of the time so that she doesn't have to say words that she knows are she's more likely to stutter upon. Shannon changes words so often that it's sometimes hard to follow what she is trying to say. There are also some rather long pauses in her speech too while she waits until she thinks she can say the next word fluently. Only a few people know that she stutters and she's never talked to anyone about it except her mom. She's constantly on guard with her speech, hoping that no one will notice the few instances of actual stuttering that she has.

Rationale

Some clients can get away with trying to hide their stuttering, but those who do go to great lengths not to let others find out. It's seems like it's their "dirty little secret." The person who stutters seeks to keep his or her secret at practically any cost. For most people who stutter covertly, the outward signs of their disfluent speech are kept to a bare minimum. In this way, they walk the line between the regular world and others who stutter. But, like any lie, soon another lie is needed to cover for the first lie, and a web of lies is soon woven.

Sometimes, the fear is worse than the stutter, and the thought of purposefully stuttering is like intentionally touching a snake to an ophidiophobic (a person with a fear of snakes). In both instances, the fear is out of proportion to the real danger. One way to get past the fear of stuttering is for the client to stutter on purpose, the thing he dreads the most. Voluntary stuttering, or pseudostuttering as it is sometimes referred to, is used with all people who stutter because almost all share a disdain and anxiety that they will stutter again and be embarrassed. But stuttering on purpose reduces the potential for ridicule because the client is doing it on purpose, rather than "something strange" happening to him. There is a difference between someone telling others that he or she stutters and having others observe his stuttering and acting as if nothing had happened. By stuttering purposefully, it is within your control and not as feared. Afterward, there is nothing more to fear because the secret has been revealed and it is now known by others.

Voluntary stutters are also used by clients who have finished therapy to reduce their fears and anxiety related to stuttering. It is important to maintain control of stuttering and sometimes stuttering on purpose "keeps it real," even for very accomplished speakers who stutter.

Description

Voluntary stutters are usually easy repetitions of a sound or syllable. They are used to reduce the fear of stuttering or by a client to disclose his stuttering in a subtle way to listeners. Stuttering voluntarily by having blocks and struggling usually does not increase the intended outcome. The volitional stuttering is most often done right at the beginning of an interaction, when the fears are the highest. The client usually says something like, "My - my - my name is Bob." The repetitions are light and easy, without signs of struggle.

Clinical Insight: For some who stutter, the fear others will find out about their stuttering is very intense. Of course, the fear that others will find out actually makes it more likely that stuttering will occur. What is significantly different is that the voluntary stuttering is under the speaker's control, rather than being involuntary.

However, despite it feeling different, the vast majority of people who stutter still find voluntary stuttering quite distasteful and most are very reluctant to do it. Therefore, it is important for the clinician lead the way and demonstrate voluntary stuttering for the client. In this way he can stand back and observe the reactions of others for himself. But don't be surprised if the client is still reluctant to try it. It is important to be able to manage fear and anxieties effectively. Not all medicines that are good for you taste good.

Instructions to the Client

Chances are great that the client may not be receptive to this activity and so the clinician needs to be firm, positive, and upbeat in her demeanor, not letting the client's reluctance influence her resolve. It is important to explain the purpose of the activity to the client so he understands the rationale behind it. Voluntary stutters help to soften the client's disdain for his stuttering. The fear of stuttering represents one of the most difficult obstacles to speaking and if the client can overcome his fear, he will encounter greater natural fluency and offer less resistance in therapy.

The clinician might instruct the client like this; *"It's important that we start chipping away at the fear and anxiety that your stuttering creates. People who stutter are very sensitive to their stuttering—in some cases overly sensitive in that it can block the path to greater success in therapy. What I'd like do to is have you stutter on purpose right at the beginning of your sentence. I think we should start with some mild, easy repetitions, just enough so that the listener will notice them, but not be alarmed. Most clients find this hard to do at first and say that they are coming to therapy so that they don't have to stutter. Most are curious why I would ask them to stutter intentionally, when they are coming to therapy for exactly the opposite reason. The answer is that the fear of stuttering creates more muscle tension than is necessary, and muscle tension increases stuttering. So, if we can reduce the fear, we will reduce the muscle tension, and reduce the stuttering."*

"So I will go first and show you what I'm looking for you to do. I'll introduce myself to a stranger outside the clinic and ask directions to the nearest shopping mall. I'd like you to watch the expression on the listener's face and my face; I intend to stutter in a way that says 'everything is okay' and not elicit much of a reaction from the listener. To do that I'll need to stutter easily and not show distress or struggle. After I'm done, we'll see how you can manage it. Let's get our coats and give it a try."

It is usually a good idea to practice in safe area like the treatment room. Afterward, the clinician and client can reflect on the activity, discussing the listener's reaction and the client's feelings about the experience. Follow up with an assignment to stutter purposefully with two people each day and discuss it again at the next session. Later, voluntary stutters can be more "dramatic" and include some struggle and secondary characteristics. Voluntary stuttering is a good beginning to transitioning into striking up a conversation about stuttering. After the client's stuttering is disclosed to the listener, he will find that there is an intellectual interest in the topic. Preparing and rehearsing a brief script about the stuttering will help the client organize his thoughts about it. To the client's surprise, the topic likely will be met with true interest and not ridicule.

Suggested Materials

Voluntary stuttering is more about courage than materials. After practicing a few times in the therapy room, the clinician might introduce a few people from the agency that the client has not met before. The clinician can "prime" them in advance so they will know how to react.

Advance Preparation

> **Client Profile**
>
> Jared is getting the feel of controlling his stuttering blocks and beginning to enjoy some control over his stuttering. His attempts still reflect some struggle behaviors, but he is making steady progress. As a result, he is not as anxious about speaking, but he needs to develop a greater skill level in managing his stuttering. Jared typically blocks on the words that he has learned are more difficult for him to say and he is very aware of them. His nervousness can be seen in very subtle ways, like taking a slight inhalation just before trying to say a feared word. He is not completely aware of this behavior, which means the fear is still too high. Even though his control of his stuttering requires more work, he is very excited and motivated by his progress.

Rationale

Stuttering modification techniques are first used as a reaction to stuttering or are employed after the stuttering block has already begun. As the client becomes more adept at using pull-outs, bounces, and the like when he begins to stutter, employing them *before* he begins to stutter will make them even more effective. For example, clients who can predict the words they will stutter on might begin to use a pull-out as they begin to articulate the word, rather than after they have started to stutter on it. In that way, the muscle tension and other maladaptive speaking behaviors are diminished straightaway and the utterance (and stuttering) is approached with less anxiety and struggle.

These advance preparations to use stuttering modifications can be used as a transition to fluency enhancing speaking techniques. At this point, the similarity is that with fluency enhancing techniques (light articulatory contacts, voice onset, etc.) is we are asking the client to do something differently before the utterance. The other stuttering modification targets are employed after the utterance is started, in response to stuttering.

Description

Select a reading passage and have the client underline the words he feels he is most likely to stutter on. Pick a stuttering modification target for the client to use (e.g., a pull out). Have the client use the pull out at the beginning of the unlined words instead of waiting for a stutter to occur. In this way, the client either avoids stuttering on the word, or significantly diminishes the strength of the disfluency by using targets in this preventive manner.

Clinical Insight: Advance preparations are a logical extension of using stuttering modification targets to gain control of stuttering. Why wait for something to happen before taking appropriate measures? If you are going outdoors and know it's cold, you would put on your coat before going outside. You don't go outdoors and then put on the coat. If you are aware that something (a stutter) is likely to happen, taking steps to prevent or minimize the outcome is a prudent action. Most clients enjoy the opportunity to ward off moments of stuttering whenever they can, so this activity will most likely be warmly welcomed. Gaining control over stuttering is a very positive empowerment.

Instructions to the Client

To get the feel of using the targets preventively, it may be helpful for the client to use the targets at the beginning of every word, instead of just ones he thinks he may have trouble on. Prepare a list of sentences for the client to read. You'll recall that reading usually is easier for the client in that he need not generate novel ideas to express, he can just read sentences aloud. *"Now that you're getting good at modifying your stuttering using these techniques, I'd like for you to try using them* before *a disfluency occurs. In that way, I think you will see that you will stutter less and if you do stutter, it will be greatly diminished from what it might otherwise have been."*

"I'd like you to read this first sentence and use the pull-out technique at the beginning of every word. Don't wait until you stutter before using the target; getting out ahead of the stutter will give you even greater control of your stuttering. It may feel and sound a little funny at first, but the important lesson to be learned is that advance preparation results in less tension. Okay, let me show you what I want you to do. 'Iiiiiii waaaaaaant toooooo buuuuuuuy aaaaaaaa neeeeeeeew waaaaaaatch.' You say the same thing and feel how much less tension there is as you speak. Keep in mind that this is not *how the final product of therapy will sound; it's just another step along the way. Okay, let's hear you do it."*

Suggested Materials

Start out reading individual sentences aloud. Having a natural break between the sentences will enable you to discuss the client's performance and draw his attention to feeling of there being less tension while speaking. After a while, have him shorten the duration of the pull-outs; enable the client to realize that shorter pull-outs sound closer to normal speech, which is the intent of therapy.

As the client becomes more adept, prepare a few topics that he can talk about for 2 or 3 minutes by himself in a monologue. This will present a greater challenge than reading. Following that, you might engage the client in conversation; again to increase the level of challenge while maintaining his target use.

Signs of Progress in Therapy

Improvements in stuttering therapy may not always be obvious. Sometimes, it is as much a matter of knowing where to look for progress as it is being able to interpret what you see. Although progress is commonly measured in the reduced frequency of disfluencies, there are many other, more subtle aspects of behavior and cognitive awareness that are indicative of positive changes in stuttering. As clinicians become more familiar with their clients and with the disorder of stuttering, signs of progress may be found along several dimensions. The list below offers some areas in which forward development may be observed.

1. **Awareness of the core features, secondary characteristics, and feelings and beliefs about stuttering.** A client's ability to accurately and objectively identify the elements of the core features of his or her stuttering and the secondary behaviors they evoke, demonstrates the emergence of greater openness and objectivity toward their stuttering. It is typical of most clients to attempt to block their awareness of their stuttering because it can be such a psychologically painful experience. Thus, growth in the objective perception of their stuttering indicates a willingness to let down the psychological defense mechanisms and be more open and objective about what is happening.

Ideally, a client should be able to quickly identify the errant components of his speech to be able to correct them on his own. Knowledge and awareness of stuttering itself is often an early goal of stuttering therapy. It's not enough for the client to recognize that "I'm stuck" or "I messed up." He needs to be able to specify the type of disfluency (block, repetition, or prolongation) he is having and identify anatomically where it happened (the vocal folds, lips, tongue, etc.). Using specific, objective terms creates an environment of objectivity in which stuttering can be discussed as an intellectual topic, rather than being a personal flaw.

2. **Changes in stuttering behaviors.** Any change in or modification to the habitual pattern of stuttering represents an opportunity to break down the pattern that has become so strongly ingrained. Changes might include being able to modify or eliminate a secondary stuttering behavior, such as loss of eye contact or head bobbing during disfluent moments or the ability to modify a core feature of stuttering, by stretching out or "bouncing" on a disfluent sound instead of blocking on it. In the beginning, any change is desirable because it reflects the ability to deviate from what has become habituated. Later, as the client finds modifying stuttering to become easier, these changes can be shaped to more closely approximate the characteristics of normal fluent speech production.

As this process progresses, the client learns that he or she can influence and later exert a degree of control over stuttering. Having some control of stuttering is empowering. Clients can then be persuaded that they can manage their stuttering in a different way, and eventually become responsible for managing their fluency. This empowerment eventually leads to less angst over stuttering and reduces muscular tension, both of which contribute to fewer instances of stuttering.

3. **Mastery of speech targets and techniques.** A core element of stuttering therapy is learning to use speech targets (speaking techniques that address the specific aspects of the client's stuttering) to minimize his stuttering and speak in a manner that maximizes

fluency. The degree to which a client can successfully demonstrate target use in progressively more difficult speaking situations is truly progress. Most of the data collection in therapy sessions serves to document the client's target use in situations structured to challenge his emerging fluency skills. However, success in using targets is not always reflected in a steady decrease in the number of disfluencies. Rather, it is more typical of this success rate to vary; sometimes greatly. The fluency improvement curve is more like following a stock on the stock market—a continuous series of ups and downs, and if you've picked a good stock, the overall direction of the stock price over time will be upward.

This variability can be frustrating for the client and clinician. But both must recognize that day to day and situation to situation changes reflect many variables, including the client's confidence, attitude, and environmental stressors. From one perspective, stuttering control can seem like someone's mood; it fluctuates day to day, even hour by hour. But looking at someone's mood over a longer period of time, you get to see the type of person they are, basically happy or unhappy. With these changes in stuttering control, a bad day is not necessarily indicative of stuttering worsening.

4. Control of stuttering moments. A person's ability to modify and gain control over their core stuttering behaviors while speaking is an indicator of their ability to control their stuttering. When involved in a moment of stuttering, many clients escalate their efforts to push through the disfluency by pushing harder, sometimes forcing the sounds out. Typically, this includes more muscular effort articulating a sound accompanied by a more forceful exhalated breath stream and sometimes a rise in intensity and pitch as well. These seem to be the client's intuitive reactions to "getting stuck." But this response serves only to strengthen the severity of stuttering. When a client then begins to ease muscular efforts, instead of increase them, in response to a disfluency, that is progress. He is now "stuttering smarter" by reacting in a way that serves to minimize the disfluencies. In time, the client can learn to negotiate disfluencies in much the same way a skier negotiates moguls on a downhill ski run.

5. Reduced fear of stuttering. Fear of stuttering adds to the client's level of tension, undermines his confidence, and his ability to effectively access speech targets. As the client discovers he can exert some control over his stuttering, he begins to worry less about his disfluencies, as he can now more adeptly work his way out of them, and thereby be less embarrassed by them. Effective therapy works to lessen the fears by learning to be more accepting of stuttering and developing a more objective attitude toward it. Therapy exercises such as stuttering on purpose can enable the client to experience stuttering in a different way, although clients usually loath it. With exposure, the client will find that when he is in control of stuttering that it is quite a different experience. When he purposefully begins the stutter, he can purposefully stop it, although at first some purposeful stuttering can become real stuttering. Nonetheless, stuttering is not as scary when it is done volitionally.

Purposeful stuttering can begin with rather effortless repetitions of an initial sound of an utterance. The clinician might well demonstrate purposeful, easy stuttering for the client and allow him to observe listener reactions. At a later time, the clinician also may wish to demonstrate purposeful stuttering of a more severe character to seed a discussion of listener reactions. Clients' typical reactions are, "There, see what it feels like when people react to your stuttering!" The clinician will indeed gain sensitivity to the client's perspective, but more importantly, it can engage the client in a discussion of how he feels in this situation. This then becomes a teaching moment; an opportunity for the clinician to help the client interpret a listener's reaction to stuttering and instruct the client in ways of managing it effectively. For "shyer" clinicians, viewing a video of someone else stuttering may also serve the same purpose. Talking about feelings and fears is the venue toward overcoming them. An initial step is to learn about the client's experiences and perceptions.

6. Target use in stressful situations. The ability to use, or attempting to use, speech techniques in increasingly more challenging speaking situations is a sign that the client is moving out of his or her comfort zone. This demonstrates the client's emerging ability to manage the fears learned from past experiences. It is common for clients to "forget" to use their targets when they are initially overwhelmed by their fears generated from stressful situations. In these instances, clinicians should watch for the trigger that precipitates the client's stuttering. Often, there is a subtle event that triggers the client's loss of control, which he is unaware of. For example, when placing a telephone call, the listener picking up can be the trigger. This signals the point when the client must begin speaking. It is hard to predict exactly how many times the phone will ring before it is answered; or maybe no one will answer and the client will need to leave a message on the machine. Consequently, this scenario can easily become the subject of great apprehension. It requires quick reactions on the part of the client, which is not his strength and does not facilitate his fluency. Being aware of the trigger can help the client focus his attention on the event and avoid his habitual means of responding: stuttering.

Learning to manage triggers is a sign of advancement that enables the client to speak more successfully by better managing his fears. Helping the client see the predictability of the sequences of his reactions to fear helps him know what to change; in the beginning, any change is positive. If you know something will happen, it is less likely to take you by surprise and thereby enables you to respond in a different way; a way that will promote speech fluency.

Also helpful in overcoming fears are repeated exposures and guided experiences. One problem overcoming speaking fears is that most situations only offer one opportunity to engage in the difficult situation. Creating repeated opportunities, such as having the client introduce himself individually to members of a group in succession affords the chance to try, try, and try again. Usually, fears begin to dissipate over attempts in rapid succession. Thus, the client may feel his anxiety decrease as he introduces himself again and again.

Also useful may be having the client stand next to you while you speak to a group. The client is instructed not to talk. This enables the client to feel the pressures of being before an audience with the security of not having to talk. Later, as the client becomes more comfortable, the clinician may have an individual conversation with the client while both stand in front of the group. Gradually, give the client more and more speaking time.

This gradual approach allows the client to move beyond his anxiety in more manageable increments until he is talking to everyone by himself. The anxieties that underlie stressful situations take time to totally overcome; in fact, even experienced people who give lectures professionally experience anxiety at the beginning of their talks, so the anxiety should not be expected to disappear. Much time is spent learning to make anxiety manageable so that the client can access his speaking targets. This skill is of critical importance, and once learned, can be generalized to most other feared speaking situations.

7. Openness of feelings. Being able to access and discuss feelings about one's self and one's stuttering are tremendously difficult obstacles for many clients. Often the feelings are so strong and so painful that clients have learned that they can function better by tucking them away and ignoring them. Over the years, these buried feelings become harder to access and clients seem numbed to the pain; which is precisely why it is so difficult to engage clients in a discussion of this topic in therapy. Clients who become evasive when asked about their feelings likely have lost the ability to access them and usually do not relish the opportunity to do so. For others, their feelings are more of a "raw nerve" or an open wound. For either type client, clinicians should not be surprised by an eventual flood of emotions pouring from the client.

Approaches to work with clients' emotions are offered in this book. Remember that the client's feelings, attitudes, and beliefs serve to create and fuel the anxiety that creates muscle tension. This, in turn, increases the frequency of stuttering. When clients begin to talk about their feelings, it opens the door for the clinician to address this side of the stuttering problem. It signals the client's willingness to bring down protective barriers and begin to attend to the emotional components of their stuttering.

8. Mastery of fluency. An ultimate goal of therapy is for the client to be able to use the stuttering modification and fluency enhancement speech techniques to manage fluent speech. Once a client feels empowered by the techniques, he still must also take responsibility to use them to make his own fluency. As the client becomes more skilled, it is reflected in his ability to manage fluency, first in nonthreatening situations, and gradually to more difficult speaking situations. Many clients complain that the fluency they are able to maintain in the clinic is much greater than in other situations at home, in school, or at work. This is typical, and although an initial frustration for many clients, it is a window into their future fluency abilities in all other situations. It also is likely that fluency will be variable at first, but then be demonstrated more consistently in the months to follow. This emerging and fragile skill demonstrates a generally upward progression, with peaks and dips of success along the way.

9. Responsibility for effecting change. At first, clients perceive themselves as a victim of their stuttering, but as the feeling of empowerment to affect fluency grows, they realize that they must assume responsibility for being fluent. Somewhat surprisingly, this is not always what clients want. Many have the expectation that stuttering will disappear and that they will just be able to speak without needing to manage or monitor their utterances. Although this may be true in the years to come, for the present, clients must look inward to create fluent speech. Some perceive that external factors are responsible for their disfluencies. Many clients feel that there is something magical about the clinic environment in which they experience far greater fluency than in other situations. The base of power from therapy comes in being able to be fluent because the client is speaking in a deliberate and controlled manner. Early in the process, just speaking spontaneously and being fluent is being "lucky," and in more stressful situations, the luck seems to run out and stuttering returns. It is imperative that clients be disciplined enough to practice volitional speaking until they master the techniques in order to form the foundation strong enough to combat inevitable relapses. When clients take responsibility for being fluent, they trust themselves instead of their luck.

10. Confidence as a communicator. Looking beyond controlling stuttering and managing fluency, many who stutter do not perceive themselves as being able to communicate effectively. Misperceptions of past experiences, a background of unsuccessful communications, and a history of ridicule over speaking attempts can serve to make people who stutter feel uncertain and ineffective in expressing their thoughts and ideas to others; or even their ability to hold others' interest when they speak. These feelings contribute to the anxiety and angst about talking beyond stuttering, often resulting in a poor self-image as a communicator.

Many who stutter measure the success of their communication primarily in terms of their fluency; *"I think the interview went well; I only stuttered twice."* Understanding and believing that fluency is not the only measure of communicative effectiveness can be a "hard sell" to many who stutter, but it is an important realization that messages do get across to the listener, whether there is stuttering involved or not. Clients who stutter are often surprised to find that their listener actually understood their message, in part because they feel so inadequate as a speaker. The feelings of incompetence and impotency that result are hard to describe. Communication is such a basic component of being human, and to fail to connect with others in this way, like everyone else does, can be very demoralizing and painful.

At a point in therapy, most clients find that they can challenge these feelings because of their new-found fluency skills. Changing one's self-image in any regard takes time. Like a person who has lost a good deal of weight, it can take time for the self-perception as being a "heavy person" to catch up to the physical reality of now being thin. When the dissonance between the thoughts of speaking poorly and the reality of being fluent dissolves, the opportunity presents itself to develop self-confidence and an improved self-image as a communicator. This may be reflected in greater poise and self-assurance in speaking situations and there being more "personality" in the client's speaking style. There may be an increased willingness to engage in speech interactions. Greater confidence usually serves to diminish anxieties, which reduces muscle tension, which reduces disfluencies. The cycle that fuels stuttering is reversed.

Sharing the Plan and Demonstrating Success

Clients can get more from therapy when they understand what they are doing, why they are doing it, and the direction therapy is leading them. Discussing the overall design and course of therapy helps the client to understand and buy into the treatment plan specifically designed for them. Understanding therapy enables the client to be a better observer and better reporter of events that transpire outside the therapy room. Similarly, clients are more likely to be motivated when they recognize the significance of small changes in their speech.

From the beginning, review the "master plan" of therapy with the client, explaining the significance of each component of their therapy. Help the client to understand your observations and thoughts about his stuttering, this is part of educating the client about stuttering and learning the specifics of his experience with stuttering.

The Clinical Teaching Paradigm

How do clients learn in therapy? What is the role of the clinician? What are the responsibilities of the client and of the clinician in the therapeutic setting?

A basic premise of stuttering therapy is for the client to learn to speak in different ways; ways that enable him or her to minimize existing stuttering and ways of speaking that better emulate the components of normally fluent speech production. The client is taught speaking techniques or *targets* that are to be practiced in progressively more challenging speaking situations and environments. Target use is complicated by the fear of stuttering and speaking anxieties, which are an integral part of the problems inherent in stuttering. Utilizing newly learned behaviors is exceedingly difficult under conditions where anxiety is present. When anxious, the common human response is to revert back to the old behavior. This phenomenon appears to happen without the client's conscious recognition. When he is asked why he did not use the new target, the response is frequently, "I guess I forgot." He intended to use the new target, but under the stress of anxiety he subconsciously reverted back to his old habit pattern.

Speech targets usually address the components of stuttering that are dysfunctional. For example, if the client's vocal folds are tightly adducted and no air is able to be escape for speech, a target will be prescribed that serves to overcome that aberrant dimension. The client learns to replace the dysfunctional speaking behavior with the new target. Although a fairly simple and straightforward undertaking, the task can be significantly complicated by the client's apprehension and fears.

The learning paradigm can be enhanced by two relatively simply strategies: anticipation and reflection. Anticipation involves directing the client's attention to what he is expected to learn. The 60 seconds it takes to describe what the client is expected to learn before starting an activity usually pays big dividends. Anyone's awareness (and therefore his learning) is heightened by being told what to expect and what to look for. Anticipation also increases the client's awareness of what he experiences. In doing so, the client's perceptions are guided or directed to specific aspects of the experience. For example, the clinician might explain to the client, "*We're going to make some phone calls and I'd like you to pay special attention to your speech just as you begin to speak, right after the person says 'hello.' I think you will see that you take a quick and deep inhalation of air that starts your speech off in the incorrect way. Let's make the first call and see if you notice what I'm talking about.*" Often, clients are not aware of some of their speaking behaviors in more stressful situations. But, by drawing attention to this specific behavior, the client becomes aware of his maladaptive reaction in the speaking situation. This is the first step in changing it. It is very unlikely that this learning would have taken place without first drawing the client's attention to it and getting him to anticipate the event. Clients often find a way to ignore information that "isn't flattering"; this is the ego's way of protecting us, shielding us from things that are painful, but true.

As a result, being made aware of those behaviors is somewhat confrontational and uncomfortable and many clients will go to great lengths to avoiding dealing with them. However, guided confrontation may be a means of overcoming those difficult aspects. Awareness is the first step. It often makes it more palatable to the client if the clinician states her comments as objectively as possible. Talk about the behaviors, not the person. You might say, "I noticed the rate of speech increased right after she answered the call," instead of, "*You* started speaking too fast right after she answered the phone." Clients are sometimes more open to clinician comments when they do not feel threatened by them or feel accused of doing something wrong, even in this subtle way. Discussing them in objective (nonpersonal) terms is one means of promoting that.

However, later, after the client is better able to discuss his behaviors more openly, using "*you* language" becomes an important ingredient of assigning responsibility to the client for his actions and behaviors. Not blame, but responsibility. Gauge the client's receptiveness to "*you* language" by his willingness to discuss his behaviors. Note how whether or not he refers to them in terms of "his stuttering." Remember also that there's an important distinction to be made between responsibility and blame for behaviors. The client is not to be *blamed* for things he feels are out of his control, but needs to be *responsible* for managing them effectively.

The clinician's role in the clinical teaching paradigm is to be a guide or a coach. Many clinicians have expressed concern that their client knows more about his stuttering than they do. This is probably true, but not just of novice clinicians. The client has spent much more time with his stuttering than the clinician and therefore are likely to know much more about it. However, their knowledge is not always correct, and there is much that every client has yet to learn about their stuttering. We see that even the best professional athletes have coaches. For example, the best tennis players have a coach. Playing tennis, the athlete could quite handily beat his coach in a game. So, what is the purpose of having a coach that is not as good a player as the professional athlete? What the coach (and in stuttering therapy, the clinician) brings to the table is the ability to see the player from a perspective that the player cannot. The coach knows the game and how to play it, but can also provide feedback to the player that the player is unable to see from his perspective on the court. And, thus, the clinician knows about stuttering, but can also offer feedback from a perspective that is not available to the client.

Giving Feedback

Many clinicians underestimate the importance of giving meaningful feedback before, during, and after a therapeutic activity. Although saying "Good job!" provides the client with general information about his performance, it falls woefully short of the potential for communicating the information necessary to be meaningful or making clinical teaching/learning truly effective. What specifically was it about the client's response that was good? Let's look at some ways to maximize the feedback to the client.

1. Giving Instructions. Instructions set the stage for what is expected of the client. They should be relatively brief, yet explain the general intent and purpose of the activity, while describing specifically what the client is expected to do. Instructions should take no more than 20 to 30 seconds to complete. Spending time covering every nuance and possible outcome is likely not working as efficiently as you can. Be succinct and respect therapy time as the *client's* time to practice and learn. If the client misunderstands the instructions, it is usually fairly simple to redirect him, and takes but a few seconds.

Begin by explaining the purpose of the activity in terms of the expectations of the client's performance, the challenges presented, and how this fits into the overall treatment plan. When clients understand the rationale and significance of what they are being asked to do, their motivation will increase and their learning will be enhanced. If the activity entails using a speech target, model the target while instructing the client. This *shows* the client what is expected of him in addition to it being explained to him. The power of modeling is hard to overestimate. Succinctly explain how the patient is to use any materials provided for the activity. Consider having the client demonstrate his understanding of what is expected on the first item of the activity. This enables the clinician to assess his comprehension and provide further instruction if necessary.

Last, inform the client of the parameters of the task on which he will be evaluated. Explain what you will be looking for him to do and what behaviors he should try to avoid. The behaviors to avoid are usually the ways the client typically produces an aspect of his speech (such as an abrupt voice onset) that we are trying to change.

2. Keep Focused. Throughout her childhood, my daughter has had several coaches while playing baseball. A few of her coaches stood out as being markedly better than the others. At batting practice, some coaches gave the instruction to "Keep your eye on the ball." After the pitch and subsequent swing, the coach provided corrective feedback on numerous things other than watching the ball; "Keep your elbow up." "Bend your knees more." "Move your weight from your back to your front foot as you swing." Although all of this feedback was indeed valid, she was left to wonder what happened to "keep your eye on the ball"? How did she perform at what the coach specifically asked her to do? As a result, children (and adults) begin to feel that they are not good at batting (or using speech targets) because they hear that they are doing so many things wrong. They infer from the coach's feedback that just about everything that they are doing is wrong and end up feeling defeated and demoralized.

The good coaches stayed on task and focused. When instructed to "Keep your eye on the ball," the coach's feedback was directed only to that specific task. Where there other things that needed to be fixed? Certainly! But staying focused on one thing at a time is the best strategy leading to success. The batter could go home feeling like he or she had done something correctly: "I kept my eye on the ball, and the coach said I did it really well!" and the children were motivated by their success.

So, even with adults, focusing on a single target is usually preferable, even with long-standing clients. Try not to allow yourself to be distracted by other behaviors that also require work. Take note of them and incorporate them into therapy at a later time, when they can receive the full focus of attention that they deserve.

3. Summarize the Client's Performance. At the conclusion of an activity, review the client's performance based on the specific parameter that he was instructed to incorporate in the activity. Then describe where his performance places him in the overall context of the treatment plan. Finally, suggest some carryover activities for the client to continue to work on outside the clinic.

It is important to establish the expectation that clients continue to practice their speech targets outside of their time in therapy sessions. Many clients are reluctant to practice their speech in the real world and wind up never completing homework assignments. This generally impacts the rate at which they progress and it is important for clients to understand that. However, it is the client's choice whether or not he will do his homework. If he chooses not to, it is still the clinician's obligation to assign homework as our role is to suggest to the client what we feel constitutes the best treatment. Like my dentist says, "*You don't have to brush all of your teeth; only the ones you want to keep.*" Working to transfer skills into environments outside the clinic enhances therapy and enables progress to be made faster. Although we cannot force clients to do what we think is best for them, we can (and should) certainly inform them of what is in their best interest.

Clients seek our help because they alone have not been able to resolve their stuttering issues. To boost your "customer satisfaction" rating, it's important to attend to the client's comments on the difficulties stuttering represents to them. Listening carefully, clients will tell you exactly what will satisfy them. With this information, it is up to the clinician to see that these goals are met or work with the client to modify his or her goals to be more reasonable in terms of potential outcomes. Discuss the client's performance in individual therapy activities in terms of the client's overarching goals and desired outcomes of their therapy.

The Structure of Individual Therapy Sessions

The following format may be a useful guide in structuring individual therapy sessions with clients who stutter. Although this format is designed specifically for stuttering therapy, it is based on principles that apply to therapy for other disorders as well. Sessions generally are composed of five basic components: a warm-up, speech activities, affective activities, summaries, and homework. The number of speech and affective components utilized in each session varies based on the needs of the client at any particular point in their therapy.

Set the tone for the session by getting started right away; remember, "make every minute matter." Your interaction usually begins in the waiting room. Get your "*chit-chatting*" done on the walk to the treatment room. As soon as you are seated in the therapy room, you might start off by reviewing the homework assignment given at the last session or begin the warm-up activity right away.

The **Warm-up activity** is a brief (5 to 10 minutes) period of speech target practice in which the clinician provides intensive cueing and feedback. This gets the client "on track" right away, enabling him to demonstrate his current level of proficiency. It also coveys the message that, "We're here to work!" Continue until the client achieves the expected performance level, equal to or better than during the last session. Speech target activities in which the client is successful at least 80% of the time or greater are usually preferable for the warm-up activity, as the client has already achieved a high level of success and the activity is more a review than learning something new. The warm-up is like starting a piano lesson by playing the scales. It reminds the piano student how to sit on the bench, how to hold their hands for playing, where to focus her attention and it gets her acclimated to the work that lies ahead.

Speech activities are directed toward practicing speech techniques (stuttering management and/or fluency enhancement) at a level that challenges the client. Clients usually work concurrently on two or three speech techniques (targets) in each session, which are set in a hierarchy of speaking situations that vary by degree of difficulty for the client. About 10 to 15 minutes are spent on each situational activity.

A challenging level is usually a speaking environment in which the client can use the target successfully 50 to 75% of the time. Clients differ in terms of situations that they find to be more and less difficult. There also is variation by the mode of speaking that the activity requires; for example reading aloud, monologues, conversations, presentations, and speaking on the phone. Most who stutter report that there are specific words, sounds, people, or situations that present more or less difficult for them. Each of these factors can contribute to the level of challenge in therapy activities. For reading activities, it may be preferable to provide material at the word, sentence, or paragraph level, depending on the client's level of functioning and the intended focus of the activity. Word-level material provides more practice opportunities to master microskills, like using light contacts specifically on plosive sounds. Sentence or paragraph materials can be more challenging and simulate the client's need to implement speech targets intermittently as needed, like in spontaneous speech.

Affective activities deal with clients' feelings, emotions, and beliefs related to their stuttering. Examples of affective therapy goals include learning to deal with stuttering more objectively, developing alternative perspectives of stuttering, improving positive self-talk, increasing self-confidence, dealing effectively with stressful speaking situations, and changing the client's self-image as a communicator. An overarching objective in working with affective aspects of stuttering is to minimize their effect on the client's bodily responses to fear and anxiety associated with speaking and stuttering.

Affective characteristics of stuttering are factors that contribute to the frequency, overt severity, and degree of handicap their stuttering presents. Work on affective therapy targets leads the client toward mentally managing his or her stuttering in more productive and less disruptive ways. Like the speech aspects of stuttering, affective issues are addressed in logical sequences, which yield measureable outcomes.

At the end of each affective activity, the clinician provides a **summary** of what was accomplished, such as the insights gained, new challenges to be addressed, or ways to better manage speaking situations. This summary is an important teaching tool as it informs the client of how the clinician views the client's performance and progress in therapy. It guides the client's work by providing both compliments and constructive criticism. In addition to describing what was accomplished in the session, the clinician may discuss the next steps in therapy, and what the client should do outside of therapy sessions to continue to improve and challenge his skills. The summary is an important, yet often underutilized, tool in clinical teaching. It provides a context for what is being learned while educating the patient about his stuttering and status in stuttering therapy.

A summary at the end of the session can similarly provide a needed perspective on that day's session. It is important for the clinician to be honest and straightforward in evaluating the client. Only discussing the "rosy side" of the patient's performance can be unfair to the client. Although most clinicians do this in an attempt to be supportive, in the end, it actually can serve to diminish the value the client places on the clinician's feedback. The most effective feedback is honest, balanced, and presented in a tactful way. This takes practice.

Most therapy activities (speech and affective activities) are 10 to 15 minutes in length. The summary following each activity should take about a minute, while clinicians typically spend about 2 minutes on the summary at the conclusion of the session. Thus, an hour-long session can include the warm-up activity, two or three therapeutic activities, and the final summary.

Homework serves several important purposes, including establishing the expectation that speech techniques should be utilized in natural contexts outside the clinic room. Clients should have something to work on *each day* to expedite their progress and facilitate carryover. Have specific tasks for the client to do at least once every day. Work with the client to detail specific times or situations in which he will complete his assignments. Trying to problem-solve with the client and including him in the planning process increases the likelihood he will complete the tasks prescribed. It's the clinician's responsibility to inform the client of what he can do independently that will enable him to progress as rapidly as he can. It remains up to the client to determine what he or she will actually do. Even though the client will not always do everything that he is advised, it's our professional responsibility to let him know what the best course of action is for him. It is then up to him to decide what to actually do. But the clinician has fulfilled her professional responsibility. It's our professional responsibility to inform the patient of the best course of action in order to improve their fluency skills most efficiently; it's the patient's decision as to what he will actually do.

Structuring a mechanism to report completed homework assignments may also encourage the client to finish his homework. Like the weekly weigh-in at Weight Watchers, having to report the results of homework assignments (particularly in a group setting) increases the pressure to actually do it. Reporting can be done via e-mail, phone messages, or completing data forms. But establishing a mechanism to report the results of their assignments increases the likelihood they will be completed.

Task Modes in Therapy

The task mode used in an activity is a variable that can be manipulated to increase or decrease the difficulty of the task for the client. The following information provides the clinician with a few insights into the use of a variety of speaking modes to promote the learning of new techniques and challenging emerging skills.

Reading

For most clients, reading is a less demanding form of oral communication than speaking as the words, lexicon, and ideas are already represented in the text to be read. However, there are individual exceptions. Some clients have reading difficulties that add to the disfluencies in their oral reading. In these instances, reading activities should be used sparingly or materials selected that are skill-appropriate. For others, written materials obviate the client's use of avoidance tactics. Substituting words for those that are perceived as being likely to be stuttered on is much easier to detect in reading than in spontaneous speech.

Reading, however, is a good starting point for most clients. Some clients are able to read aloud with significantly less disfluency. For these clients, it is suggested that short articles be selected, followed by a discussion or summary of what has been read. One idea is to use "Dear Abby," "Ask Ann Landers," or "Miss Manners" articles from the newspaper. Paste the letter on one side of an index card and the columnist's answer on the other side. Have the client read the letter aloud, and then provide his own answer. Finally, have the client read the columnist's response aloud. This blend of reading, speaking, and reading again can be used to flow from a "strength" (reading) to a "challenge" (conversation) and back to a "strength" again. This should promote the successful use of the target in more difficult modes.

For clients who have disfluencies reading, having a prepared text offers the clinician the advantage of knowing what the client is attempting to say, making it easier to provide instruction and feedback. Reading can be used to identify and analyze disfluencies and as an activity to implement speaking targets. Clinicians are encouraged to give clients feedback immediately while they read, stopping them when necessary. Clinicians should not wait until the client is finished reading a whole paragraph before instructing them in ways of improving their use of the speaking technique or to give them feedback. Many clinicians have a tendency to advise clients on many types of errors they make. It is better to focus on one speech target at a time, rather than mix too many together.

Monologue

Although some clients are very talkative, others are exceedingly quiet and it can be difficult to get them to talk. Many adults who stutter have not had much positive experience talking and are very comfortable being verbally introverted. Adolescents, too, may prove to be very reluctant to speak. For others, their stuttering is more of an annoyance or a frustration, hindering them from saying the many things they want to communicate. For this type of client, target use may be yet a further encumbrance and it seems that their message is more important than learning to improve their stuttering. With these profiles in mind, using a monologue task may or may not be appropriate for each individual client.

For clients who are reluctant to speak, the clinician should not ask questions which can be answered with "yes" or "no." A picture description task or having the client give directions to a local landmark may be a more effective strategy in getting him to talk. Learning to become a better conversationalist may be yet another goal in therapy.

Clients reluctant to volunteer a sufficient number of responses might better be presented reading tasks. Clients who are more verbose may require frequent interruption and direction. Some clients do not always discern that, in therapy, clinicians are more interested in "how" things are said, than "what" is said. (In counseling sessions, however, just the opposite is true.) Inexperienced clinicians are often reluctant to interrupt a client before they complete the entirety what they are saying. However, a great deal of therapy time is lost by allowing the client to stutter on word after word, not attempting to use any of his targets. Intrinsically, clients understand that it is the clinician's job to monitor his or her speech and provide feedback. As clinicians mature, they learn to diplomatically stop the client, give instruction or feedback, and resume the monologue with better target use. The objective of the task should be foremost in the clinician's mind in managing a client's speaking behaviors; maximize the number of successes in each task. The length of monologue tasks is also an important variable; begin short, expanding the length of the monologue to correspond with the client's rate of success.

Conversation

The conversation mode is usually a more demanding task, as it allows little time to formulate and reply to the listener's verbal response. As such, managing a slower rate of communication can be a vital component to the client's success. Emotional topics such as abortion or gun control may evoke feelings so strong that they compete with the client's ability to self-monitor and use speech targets. Nonetheless, such topics provide challenges as clients become more skillful at using targets.

Conversations enable the clinician to model targeted techniques while conversing with the client. Later, the clinician may use hurrying, disinterest, inattention, and interruptions to challenge more advanced clients.

Conversation is also a mode that can be used to transition from the clinic to the real world. Engaging strangers in conversations, speaking with co-workers, and conversing at social gatherings are activities that many people who stutter find stressful and challenging. As such, group therapy may pave the way toward transitioning to real-world experiences. These real-world encounters frequently represent a greater challenge and as such, clients initially regress in their skill level.

Presentations

One of the most common stresses for virtually everyone, whether a person who stutters or not, is giving presentations. A presentation is most like an extended, prepared, rehearsed, and formal monologue. In my experience, a therapy assignment to prepare a presentation at the next treatment session often results in an excuse for not completing it; "I forgot." or "I didn't have time." This is most often a translation of, "I was too frightened to do it." But, when the client needs to do a presentation at work or at school, he is suddenly "highly motivated" to work on his talk. Unfortunately, the big presentation is usually the next day or in a few days, leaving inadequate time for any real constructive improvements to be made. It is at the clinician's discretion whether to try to work on it or not. Attempting to prepare the client for something far beyond his current skill level most often has little to no impact and the client's feelings of "this doesn't work" may be reinforced. It may be more appropriate for the clinician to say, "This requires much more work than we can do in the few days left. We can, however, begin today to prepare for the next talk you will need to give, but there is very little we can accomplish right now for your talk tomorrow. We need to learn from this experience and devote more time to preparing for future speaking occasions that will arise."

Spontaneous presentations are a very good as a group therapy activity. As such, one of the goals is to become more relaxed while in the role of the speaker and the center of attention. Presentations should be long enough to have the client experience the anxiety and also to feel it dissipate while standing before the group. Learning to be more comfortable in the role of the speaker comes from multiple opportunities, in several different environments. Moving outside of the client's comfort zone promotes a feeling of fear, excitement, and opportunity; the key ingredients of change and improvement.

Telephone Calls

Clients who stutter commonly fear speaking on the phone. Many express the concern that all the attention is focused on their speech because the listener can't see them and doesn't know what is going on. This attention increases the client's fear and tension, which usually increases their stuttering.

Another significant issue in using the phone is the time it takes the client to initiate his speech. Listeners can be very impatient when it appears that no one is on the other end of the phone or the thought that it is a "prank call." Listeners wait only a few seconds before hanging up, an experience the client has likely encountered numerous times before. This time pressure typically is very difficult for people who stutter and usually serves to precipitate stuttering blocks. Under this pressure, the client seldom realizes how much his speaking pattern changes when attempting to use the telephone. Just the thought of making a call stirs emotions and consequently physical changes in the process of speaking.

Thus, telephone calls often begin with desensitization tasks; stuttering voluntarily to a known listener while asking the store's hours. As the client becomes less fearful and better able to initiate voice, continued practice will result in smoother, softer initiation of speech. Attention needs to be focused on the changes made to the normal, fluent speaking process while practicing phone calls. Often, the client's breaths become shorter and more rapid when speaking on the phone. Typically, clients take a deep gasp of air immediately before trying to phonate, almost ensuring they will block. As awareness builds, clients begin to see the pattern that leads them into almost certain stuttering. With the clinician's guidance, they begin to better implement their speech targets and eventually overcome their difficulty speaking on the phone. For most, it is a long and difficult struggle, filled with successes and failures. Persistence is required to overcome speaking fear on the phone.

In General

Talking with your client enables you to begin to learn their feared situations, words, and sounds. In the vast majority of cases, the client's pattern of speaking changes dramatically in these feared situations, most often without their complete awareness. The clinician should not take the client's reassurances that particular situations do not present difficulty for them, as some clients attempt to mask their fears with such bravado. A few actual telephone calls will reveal the client's actual abilities. Someone who doesn't find telephoning difficult shouldn't mind making a few calls.

Sample Therapy Session

Treatment sessions have a number of common goals and themes. The activities used to challenge the client are determined by his performance level and progress in therapy to date. Subsequent to the initial treatment meeting, each session contains elements of information gathering, review of speech targets, progressive speaking challenges, reflection, a summary, and homework. Good clinicians continually learn new things about their clients in each session. Probing and questioning the client to determine his knowledge, feelings, thoughts, and beliefs about aspects of his stuttering is an ongoing process. The clinician might try to construct a model of the client's perspectives on his stuttering to better understand, support, and motivate him in therapy. Engaging the client in conversation about stuttering often does not feel like therapy to clinicians new to stuttering, but these counseling conversations are really key to being effective in addressing the client's needs. As the clinician-client relationship develops over time, this information usually becomes easier to obtain as trust in the relationship grows.

It is important to set a supportive, enthusiastic work tone for each session; after all, each minute of therapy matters. Sessions might begin with a minute's discussion of the client's speech since the last session and a review of his homework. The unfortunate, but common, reality is that clients often do not practice implementing their targets outside the clinic setting. As a result, it is important to ensure that the client knows the targets and can demonstrate their correct usage when he returns to the next session. Reading is usually the therapy first activity of each session and an opportunity for the client to demonstrate that he is using the speech targets properly. This affords the clinician the chance to modify his responses that are not 100% correct. When the client demonstrates correct target use for 1 full minute, the clinician can summarize the client's performance in a few sentences and the second activity can be initiated. Again, the objective of this warm-up activity is to establish correct speech target usage and to correct it if necessary.

The second activity might be a conversation in which the client uses one of his speech targets. At the beginning, the clinician models the targets as part of instructing and demonstrating the desired response for the client; but the modeling decreases as the client demonstrates successes. Specific feedback regarding the client's accuracy and quality of targets used is intense during the first minute of the conversation, but then fades as the client's successful use of targets continues. At the beginning of the activity, corrective or affirming feedback is provided at least every 30 seconds. Following that, sporadic feedback is offered as long as the client continues to successfully use the target.

As the client's accuracy level increases in conversation, the speaking situation can be made more challenging. Speaking to a stranger, making introductions to others, giving a timed presentation or monologue, or making phone calls can often serve to raise the level of challenge. It is important that sessions contain activities in which the client struggles, as well as activities in which he will be highly successful. Growth in therapy comes from the struggling; but struggling to just the right degree. Struggling indicates that the client is working just beyond his capacity to be successful and in an area in which he is able to grow. Analogously, if you play tennis against someone who is just a little bit better than you, you will improve faster than playing against someone who is your equal or not quite as good as you are. Without challenges, clients do not improve as quickly as they are able. It is important to reflect upon and discuss the client's performance in challenging situations as a means of stimulating his growth and motivating his future successes. This presents the opportunity for the clinician to influence the client's perception of the activity, effectively teaching him how to interpret what happened and how to change it in subsequent attempts. Often, a client's perception of an event is skewed by his feelings about stuttering. He may sincerely feel that he tried to use a speech target, but is not aware of how and when he went askew. This teaching moment is a vital part of therapy. The clinician's objective observations and interpretations help shape the client's perceptions and teach him how to see his stuttering and how to change. This feedback is often overlooked by clinicians, missing an important opportunity. Guiding the client's reflections in the treatment room also helps him to alter his perceptions of stuttering outside of therapy.

A third activity might incorporate something to address the client's feelings and emotions. This typically takes the form of a discussion of a topic relating to stuttering or testing out his beliefs about stuttering in the real world. It would be ideal if the client used his speech targets during this discussion, but it is not absolutely necessary. As most clients find discussing their feelings about stuttering difficult enough, using speech targets may represented an added encumbrance and thereby serve to inhibit the conversation.

Staying focused on the goal of the activity, bringing out feelings and emotions, should take precedence over target use. It may, however, be of interest to the clinician to see how the client chooses to manage his fluency in this situation.

Discussion topics might include how to make a listener feel comfortable with the client's stuttering, how to bring up the topic of stuttering in a conversation with a friend, how to handle disfluencies during a job interview or on a date, or whether to leave a message on an answering machine or hang up. The outcome of the discussion is improved when the clinician sets the topic and has specific points she wishes to arise from the discussion, such as how bringing up the topic of stuttering when meeting someone new can serve to put both the client and the listener at greater ease. Maximize the effectiveness of the discussion by having the lessons you would like the client to gain from the activity preplanned with your points written out. You also might have some reading materials available for the client to take home to stimulate further thoughts on the topic.

At the end of each activity and at the end of each therapy session, the clinician should summarize the important points which stemmed from the day's appointment. Often, clients benefit much more from having the events and their performance interpreted for them, highlighting the clinician's agenda and the client's in the accomplishments session. The clinician should detail the client's accomplishments during the session and put them in the perspective of the overall treatment plan, thus updating the client as to their current status and what lies ahead for them.

Finally, homework is assigned that includes at least one thing for the client to do each day to help him generalize his skills using targets to environments outside of the therapy room. Homework might also direct the client to opportunities to test out some of his beliefs about stuttering at work, school or at home. It usually is prudent for the client to participate in determining how and when the homework activities will be done, because if he is assigned something that he feels is too difficult or too risky, he will not do it. It is also helpful to incorporate a means for the client to report back on his assignments during the week. It's hard to know if you are losing weight if you never weigh yourself on a scale. When the client needs to report back on his performance, it increases the likelihood that he will do it. Reporting daily via e-mail can be a useful means of communicating activities, problems encountered, and the client's thoughts on his work.

Early on in the course of treatment, more attention is focused on speaking activities, learning to modify stuttering moments, and incorporate fluency-enhancing speaking behaviors. As therapy progresses, feelings and emotions activities are introduced and eventually become the larger component of treatment sessions and homework activities.

Clients usually benefit from having two or three general themes (or slogans) which are used consistently throughout the course of therapy. Phrases such as, "*Think before you begin to speak*" or "*Get off to a good start*" provide catchphrases that the client will say to himself in other situations. These slogans help the client to understand what is important about his therapy and the purpose or directions of his work. The clinician's work also seems to be more focused to the client and therapy might not seem so overwhelming. He will find comfort in the themes and see consistency in the clinician's work.

Sample Lesson Plan

Table 3–2 presents the treatment plan for a typical session of stuttering therapy.

Organizations and Support Groups

People who stutter can learn a great deal by talking with one another. Many adults who stutter have not met or have not talked with anyone else who stutters. Remember that stuttering is typically not something the person who stutters has enjoyed talking about; in fact it is commonly attempted to be concealed. In that regard, stuttering can be quite isolating. The PWS does not want to discuss his stuttering and it consequently becomes inappropriate for others to bring it up. Most of the client's experience has come in being ridiculed about his speech, so it is natural that he try not to disclose it. Added to that, many who stutter are exceedingly uncomfortable with the stuttered speech of others because it brings up feelings about their own stuttering. However, group therapy or support groups for those who stutter are very effective venues to bring people together to talk about stuttering in a safe and very accepting way. Organizations such as the National Stuttering Association (http://www.westutter.org) and Friends (http://www.friendswhostutter.org) offer support groups and conferences that address the needs of people who stutter. Learning that others are going through many of the same experiences can be very therapeutic. Being about to talk about stuttering with others who understand the experience is a tremendous relief. Learning how others handle their speech and speaking situations can be motivational. It is hard to overstate the potential benefits of these organizations to people of all ages who stutter and to parents of children who stutter.

Table 3–2. Sample Lesson Plan

Activity	Goal	Behavioral Objective
Warm-Up: Speech Activity	Speech target use in reading	The client will read an article about the Pittsburgh Penguins using slow rate with 90% accuracy.
Two: Speech Activity	Speech target use in conversation	While discussing the upcoming hockey season, the client will use slow rate with 75% accuracy.
Three: Affective Activity	Identify and objectively describe disfluencies	Watching a video of himself in conversation, the client will identify 85% of the instances of stuttering and categorize the type of disfluency with 90% accuracy.
Four: Affective Activity	Identifying bodily affects of fear and anxiety of stuttering	Preparing to make a phone call, the client will identify and describe tension in two parts of his body and two thoughts about making calls.
Homework: Speech Activity	Speech target use in reading	During dinner each evening, the client will select a brief article from the newspaper and read it to his family using slow rate.

Reference

Van Riper, C., & Erickson, R. (1996). *Speech correction: An introduction to speech pathology and audiology* (9th ed.). Needham, MA: Allyn and Bacon.

CHAPTER

4

Activities for Stuttering Therapy

Stuttering therapy addresses two sides of the problem: the speech aspects and the client's feelings, emotions, attitudes, and beliefs about his stuttering. Both aspects require activities to afford the client opportunities to practice using his speaking targets and opportunities to explore his feelings and attempt to modify them.

Most clinicians are better experienced working with the speech aspects of communication disorders like stuttering. Many, at first, find it difficult to work with the other side of stuttering—the counseling aspects. But the two are intimately intertwined and a successful outcome requires work in both areas.

Stuttering is an interesting disorder to work with because it requires that a trusting relationship or bond be formed between the client and clinician. The clinician must learn to become a good listener to encourage the client to discuss his perceptions of his stuttering; a strong motivator to push the client into situations he finds challenging; and an honest evaluator of his work, performance, and efforts. Embrace those qualities and you, and your client, will be successful.

This chapter offers examples of ways to approach various aspects of speech target use and the emotive components of stuttering problems in therapy.

Chapter Outline

Introduction

Activities are the lifeblood of every therapy program for any communicative disorder. In stuttering therapy, activities have dual purposes. Some focus on providing opportunities for clients to practice using their speech targets; others offer a means to address the client's feelings, emotions, and beliefs that have developed in response to their stuttering. These counseling-oriented activities are selected to match the different individual needs of adults who stutter and parents of children who stutter. Some discussion of these two related goals is warranted before beginning to plan therapy activities.

Speech Activities

Speech activities intend to provide opportunities for a client to talk, giving him a context and a purpose to practice using the speech targets that are a part of his therapy program. Providing a proper context for an activity is a vital part of making therapy effective. For example, sometimes adult clients might be asked to read a children's book. The intent in selecting the children's book for the activity is primarily for the client to practice reading slowly and with greater intonation and inflection. But, out of context, asking an adult client to read a children's book may strike the client as being demeaning. The client's initial reaction might be, *"Does she think I can't read very well? Does she think I'm that dumb?"* But by providing a context for the activity in which the client, in real life, might actually be called upon to do will change the client's attitude and perspective. The clinician might say, *"Imagine your sister has asked you to watch her 4-year-old daughter for a couple hours while she goes out shopping. You could entertain the child by reading her a story. Good storytellers try to read in a way that allows the child to paint a picture of the words being read in their head so they can imagine what is happening. So, I'd like you to read this story about the tortoise and the hare very slowly, using more intonation and inflection that you might ordinarily use. That will help stimulate the child's imagination, understanding, and enjoyment of the story. Okay, let's begin."* Note how the context helps the client envision the therapy activity in a real-life application. He can imagine reading to a 4-year-old and will not think the clinician is discrediting his reading ability or intelligence. Establishing a context enables the client to buy into the activity and see its value beyond the therapy room.

Although therapy begins in the treatment room, the whole point is to enable the client to use his targets in the real world. As such, activities are designed to simulate, replicate, and incorporate the client's communicative environments outside of the clinical setting, while providing a safe, supportive context for his success and challenging his emerging skills. Clinicians also need to provide an extension of therapy activities into the client's other environments. Having the client tell his spouse, roommate, or friend about what he is working on in therapy and recruiting their help in practicing his skills might be a first step in making this transition. Parents of children who stutter might replicate some therapy activities in the home. Be prepared to discuss with the client how and when they can transition treatment room activities into the rest of their world.

The design of therapy also needs to respect the client's hierarchy of situational difficulties to gauge the degree of challenge for the client. Working with the client, the clinician helps to order the degree of perceived difficulty various situations present to him. In this way, the hierarchy provides a guide in making activities progressively more challenging for the client. Typically, activities begin in easier contexts and work their way through situations that are progressively more challenging. For most clients, speaking alone by themselves presents a very low level of challenge or threat. Part of the initial goal of therapy is to provide an understanding, safe, and protected workplace for the client to practice his speech targets. Speaking in a quiet therapy room with the clinician may be more difficult for the client than speaking alone by himself, but it typically is the physical location that is the starting point for an activity.

In addition to the physical location, several categories of circumstances can create challenges for clients that need to be explored in developing the hierarchy for therapy. These may include:

- specific words or sounds
- particular people or roles (such as parents, authority figures, or girls!)
- situations such as asking questions in meetings, introducing oneself, interviewing, making phone calls, socializing at parties, asking a clerk for help, giving a presentation (public speaking), testifying in court, ordering in a restaurant, and so on.

Client Profile

David recently became concerned that he was having difficulty speaking when some of his second grade classmates made fun of him. He quickly became aware that he struggled to say words which began with /f/ and /s/ sounds. In anticipation of "getting stuck" on these sounds, David tried using more force at the beginning of these words. Unfortunately, this strategy only made his problem worse and it grew even more worrisome for him. And now he was beginning to have trouble saying other words too, like his name.

David is an example of how a person's natural reaction (using more force to articulate a sound or word) only serves to make the problem worse. It is ironic that, even though these attempts are unsuccessful, people who stutter persist in using them. What David needs is another strategy; perhaps a light articulatory contact or a pull-out to change his stuttering pattern by providing him with functional tools to move beyond his stutters. Using speech techniques and practice on targeted sounds will enable David to develop a successful strategy to make these sounds fluently. With repeated practice, his fears of stuttering on these sounds will diminish as his confidence in the techniques grows.

The clinician develops a list of challenges and helps the client order them in terms of the degree of difficulty they represent. The list becomes the clinician's guide toward ordering the structure and context of therapy activities to challenge the client in a deliberate, controlled manner, without grossly exceeding his threshold of failure.

Client Profile

Jason is very self-conscious about talking in class, especially in the high school's biology class. His teacher, Mr. Sanders, has high expectations for students in his classes and requires them to answer questions in class quickly; especially when the questions are about the homework assigned the night before. Mr. Sanders sometimes seems a bit curt, but he earnestly wants his students to be prepared to compete in their classes in college next year. This pressure really affects Jason's fluency. When called on, even though he knows the answer, he often says he doesn't know, just so he won't stutter.

In Jason's case, starting off using targets in Mr. Sander's class will likely be too great a challenge and he will probably struggle and be unsuccessful, only reinforcing his current feelings and insecurities. He might begin by answering or asking questions in another class, one he perceives to be less threatening. With less stress, his chances of being successful are greater. It also may be helpful to make the teacher aware of the situation and suggest ways in which they can help the student succeed. For example, instead of calling on the student by surprise: *"What is the cube root of 16? Jason!"*—a teacher can call on the student first, pose the question, and then talk a bit more before requesting the answer. For example, *"Jason, problem number 3 in last night's homework required you to calculate the cube root of 16. You recall that the process of calculating cube root is much like that of long division; unless you use a calculator, of course! Jason, what answer did you get for number 3?"* This strategy minimizes the element of "surprise," allowing Jason to collect himself a bit and think about his speech targets before he has to answer. It also maintains the goal of the teacher: preparing students to be able articulate their thoughts and ideas when put on the spot. Both Jason and the speech pathologist should talk with teachers beforehand, so that everyone is aware of the goals and expectations.

It usually is beneficial to offer different levels of hierarchical challenges to the client concurrently. For example, the client may be presented activities at several levels in the same session, with the expectation that his performance level will be higher in the situations he has identified as *less threatening* and poorer in those considered to be *more challenging*. Thus, an initial part of an activity might be making phone calls to the clinician in another room. The next activity (at a more challenging level) in the same session would then be to call Wal-Mart to ask how late they are open. An advantage of this "spiraling" approach is that there is not a dramatic shift at a single point in therapy. He goes from an activity with a relatively high success level immediately into a more challenging activity that tests his emerging skills. One hopes there will be a degree of carryover from one to the next. The client consistently is introduced to harder situations throughout his therapy, cushioning the impact of transitions to bigger challenges. Trying something for the first time usually represents a big hurdle. With repeated practice, these hurdles become less onerous.

Experienced clinicians anticipate that there will be variability in their client's performance in any activity; it's a hallmark of working with stuttering. Performance may vary within a session or from one session to the next. Clinicians and clients should not be discouraged by these fluctuations; they are just a part of stuttering. When a client begins to exceed a 90% success rate in an activity, therapy time may be better spent on something more challenging that will enable the client to grow more in the skill. Activities in which the client's performance level is high also make good transfer activities for the client to practice in other environments outside of the clinic.

Client Profile

Kristin "freezes up" when meeting new people; she gets really anxious that she will stutter and rushes her speech, often leading her into a stuttering block. As a result, she shies away situations in which she might have to introduce herself. When such a situation arises, she sometimes awkwardly excuses herself very quickly before she has to say her name and then doesn't return. People have started to think Kristin's behaviors are strange and they don't understand what her problem is; so they tend not to include her in social events and outings.

As her peers represent a significant challenge for Kristin, she might try a change of venue. Coming from a good family, she does have good social skills, but her speech just prevents her from demonstrating them. A change of venue might enable her to be less anxious and less tense. Working with her speech pathologist or life skills teacher at her school, perhaps Kristin could help other students with challenges acquire better social skills, like introducing themselves. For example, many children with autism or children with intellectual challenges benefit from learning and practicing social skills, like making introductions. As the teacher's assistant, Kristin might find her role less threatening and benefit from some valuable practice time herself, and at the same time, be helping these other students.

Emotive Activities

Of the two parts of stuttering therapy, addressing the emotional needs of clients is by far the more challenging, and usually less familiar to clinicians. At its base, work in this area requires an understanding of the culture of stuttering. Involvement in support groups for persons who stutter can be an excellent resource for developing an understanding of the feelings common among people who stutter. It is important to remember that each person has his or her own unique experience with stuttering and therefore it would not be prudent to make assumptions that every client has the same thoughts, ideas, and beliefs about his stuttering. As a consequence, the clinician should discuss the parameters of each client's experience at some length to learn about their history and understand their perspectives on their difficulties. You can be more effective if you know how your client thinks.

Language Use in Conversations About Stuttering

Your word choice when talking about stuttering can be the difference between making a connection with a client and alienating him. A common mistake (of clinicians who do not themselves stutter) is try to relate to the client by saying something like, *"That's okay; I stutter sometimes too."* Clients are generally very sensitive to the fact that their speech (and in this case, their stuttering) is very different from the clinician's. To the client, these well-intended words demonstrate that the clinician does not really understand stuttering if she thinks her speech miscues are the same as stuttering. Instead, it generally is wiser just to listen and ask the client questions about what the experience has been like for him. Another approach is to relate the experiences of other people you know who stutter. For example, *"Many of the other clients that I work with who stutter have expressed experiences and feelings very similar to what you are telling me."*

Remember too that people who stutter want to be thought of as being just like everyone else, yet inside they feel different because of their speech. Using the "language of we," instead of referencing people who stutter as being different, can be an important demonstration of unity and understanding which works toward building the client's trust. Referring to people who stutter using expressions such as "you people" or "people with your condition" most likely will alienate the client. Adopt the philosophy of thinking that people who stutter are indeed just like everyone else; because everyone else has problems they deal with too. It may not be stuttering, but everyone has their own burden to bear, yet inside we are all more alike than we are different. If you interact with your client as though he is a friend with a problem, the language that you use in speaking with him will come out without much extra thought or effort.

Attempting to be politically correct, many clinicians (including this author) have tiptoed around talking about stuttering directly, trying not to use references that might imply that stuttered speech is in some way bad, undesirable, or wrong. But some clients refer to their own stuttered speech as having "messed up," "doing badly," or "having awful speech." This terminology reflects the client's emotions about their stuttering; the way they really feel about it. Their choice of words belies their feelings. Be cautious not to "buy into" their feelings. But instead of openly disagreeing with them by saying things like, *"You shouldn't feel that way about it,"* or *"Everybody messes up now and then,"* show the client how you think about it by using honest, objective terms, rather than demeaning, judgmental labels. *"I noticed three disfluencies when you spoke,"* or *"I didn't think that the block took away from getting your message across."* These statements acknowledge the stuttering but do not make judgments about it. Being direct and truthful is important. Trying to smooth over an incident while attempting to make the client feel better can result in losing credibility. The client is painfully aware of what happened and denying it or making light of it will not make the clinician seem competent or creditable. Be supportive and respectful by being truthful, acknowledging what is obvious to everyone in an objective way.

Saying, *"It's okay to stutter"* can be a confusing and conflicting message to the client. From the client's life experiences, his world has told him that stuttering is different, and different in a socially undesirable way. Saying it's okay does not make it okay and most clients are not swayed by the clinician's attempts at encouragement anyhow. Perhaps, the real meaning of the phrase is that *people* who stutter are okay. They are not really different from everyone else and the problems that befall their lives. Another interpretation is that "Your stuttering doesn't bother me" or "It's okay *with me* if you stutter." From yet another perspective, once a listener gets past the surprise of learning that their communication partner stutters and begins to treat him like anyone else, they will have then shown that "it's okay to stutter." Some clients interpret the message as being defeatist; meaning "you better get used to your stuttering because it's not going to change." But the conflict remains; even if stuttering is okay with others, it's not okay with the client. If it was okay, why would he be coming to therapy? Trying to convince him that his stuttering somehow is not a problem may become an obstacle in your relationship with the client.

Emotive activities address the feelings, attitudes, emotions, and beliefs held about stuttering. Although each client differs, most often people who stutter feel badly about their speaking abilities, and sometimes badly about themselves as well. For the majority of their lives, others have been overtly and covertly critical of their speech. As a consequence, most clients who stutter are hypersensitive about speaking and overly aware of their disfluencies. It is human nature for a person to try to hide what they think is "wrong" with them, especially when others continuously point to these same flaws.

Emotive therapeutic activities have numerous overall objectives. The specific needs of each client vary, but in general they include the following:

- building a knowledge base about stuttering
- managing the effects of nervousness and anxiety
- reducing fears of speaking and stuttering
- accepting stuttering

- overcoming avoidances
- negotiating difficult speaking situations
- exploring feelings and beliefs about stuttering
- assessing the impact of stuttering
- building speaking confidence
- constructing a new, positive self-concept as a communicator.

Many of these objectives are interrelated, but the point of emotive activities is to address the consequences of stuttering, which tend not to disappear completely, even after the client learns to control his stuttering behaviors.

Fear and Anxiety

Fear, anxiety, apprehension, and worry feed the overt symptoms of stuttering; they serve to precipitate instances of the underlying physiologic condition. These fear-based emotions often have rather dramatic effects on the body too. Not only does fear result in physical shakiness, muscular tension, and increased heart rate, but there are "mental" symptoms of fear too. Among them are a certain edginess and hypervigilance as the brain attempts to guard against danger. This hyperreactive state is quick to identify threats, but not as adept at discriminating real threats from imagined ones. In therapy, this hyperreactiveness can be a serious impediment to progress. Learning a new behavior in the face of anxiety is a tremendous challenge. Under these difficult circumstances, the client's old (maladaptive) habitual behaviors are easily triggered and it is hard for the client to explain why he was unable to implement a newly learned behavior. As a result, these negative emotions can also breed a sense of hopelessness and defeat as they can be so very difficult to manage.

The pattern of behaviors that develops is easily generalized; eventually any potential speaking situation generates anxiety. Some who stutter start to worry about a speaking situation months in advance of the actual presentation. Frequently, college students who stutter begin worrying the first day of class about being assigned to give a presentation at the very end of the semester. For most, even sensing their own anxiety can trigger memories of past embarrassing instances of stuttering, which then result in muscular tension at present. If the situation is left unchecked, stuttering almost certainly will become a self-fulfilling prophecy. The process seems to happen automatically and the individual feels that it is out of his control. To be able to move beyond it, the client needs to become aware of this cycle and intentionally interrupt it.

A first step is to work with the client to build his awareness of the components of his habitual response pattern to his fears. An activity in which the clinician and client watch a video of the client together can be both informative and instructive. The client and clinician work together to identify, describe, and determine the logic behind what happens when the sequence of stuttering is initiated. A trigger is an event that sets off the emotional

Client Profile

An unsettling feeling passed through Tim's body the moment he learned that doing a presentation was a requirement of a class he needed to graduate as an Engineering major. As the instructor spoke in front of the class, the only thing going through Tim's mind was how embarrassing it was going to be to stutter in front of his classmates. He had managed to talk as little as possible in his classes so far, and even selected engineering partially because he wouldn't need to interact much with future clients. But now his biggest fear was on the horizon and even though the presentation wouldn't be for several months, he was already thinking of ways he might be able to get out of doing it. He'd need to think a lot more and then maybe email the instructor to see if there was a way to get out of doing this presentation assignment. His high school teachers had allowed him to do presentations alone without the other students present, but Tim didn't think this would work in college. He was already panicking. Maybe he could work in a group and do the research whereas others did the actual presentation—the professor might buy that?! He was happy to do all of the work; just so he didn't have to present.

Sitting there in class engrossed in his worrisome thoughts, the next thing Tim realized was that everyone was staring at him waiting for him to say something. While thinking about the presentation, the instructor had called on him to introduce himself and explain what he wanted to learn from the course. Tim just sat there frozen in terror, unable to say or do anything. It was one of his worst moments in his college career; even worse than all of the things he could remember happening in high school that flashed through his mind as he just sat there at his seat, feeling stupid.

or physical chain reaction behaviors. For example, when making a phone call, it may be when the other party picks up and says "*hello*" that serves to first trigger the client's stuttering behaviors. Or, in another situation, the trigger may be as people gather for a meeting and begin to introduce themselves to the group. Or it may be when the client hears his name when he is called on to answer in class. For most events, there is a specific event that ignites or triggers the client's fear-based emotions. An initial step toward defusing it is to become aware of it in advance and then make appropriate accommodations to deal with it effectively by employing the appropriate speech target proactively.

Client Profile

Scott has trouble accepting his stuttering. It is such an embarrassment at work that he never answers the telephone when he gets calls, letting it go to voice mail. When the phone rings it startles him, sending him into immediate panic. When he tries to answer a call, nothing comes out. First, he takes a very rapid gasp of air and then his vocal folds "lock up" tightly and no sounds come out; he can't even breathe. The same thing always happens over and over again with every call.

With so much fear and anxiety, Scott is only aware that he can't talk and how embarrassed he feels. In this state, it is unlikely that he is aware of the things he is unintentionally doing that contribute to the difficulty. The deep gasp for air when starting to talk goes unnoticed because of the fear. His attempts to then force the first sound out creates so much muscular tension as to actually prevent the vocal folds from being able to vibrate. Too often, bringing these behaviors to the client's attention does little to change them. The fear is too great and the client continually reverts to his old habitual behavior. Making a video recording of the client answering a phone call can help him to see these behaviors for himself. This often is a painful experience; but it can be very motivating and effective in facilitating behavioral changes. Have the client watch the video three or four times, instructing him to watch the key elements that deviate from the normal speaking process. For Scott, being told to look for the rapid gasp of air followed by the forceful adduction of the vocal folds will ensure that he gets the message. Have the client do some negative practice; imitating his "old pattern" of answering the phone, then demonstrating a more productive manner of speaking.

Managing the Body's Response to Fear and Anxiety

A discussion of the body's normal reactions to a fear stimulus is a good starting place. The client's age and education should be considered in determining the depth of the discussion. The exchange might go something like this:

> *"People are 'hardwired' to respond to dangers in their environment; it is part of our survival instinct. This 'fight or flight' response is how we are protected from dangers, both physical and psychological ones. When something triggers a danger signal our brain responds by preparing the body to either combat or flee from the threat. In either regard, chemicals are emitted in the brain, which affect the body in several ways. Our heart rate increases,*

> *we breath more rapidly, blood flow increases especially to large muscle groups, we start to perspire, the digestive process slows down (often feeling like butterflies in the stomach), our sensory acuity is heightened, and our mental flexibility diminishes (when you're really scared it hard to even recall factual information like your own name). These changes are all in preparation to fight or flee from the danger. We are focused totally on the dangerous situation at hand."*

"What do you notice when your body responds to fears and anxiety?" (Engage the client in a self-analysis of his bodily responses to fears. Include some of your observations and ask questions to stimulate the client's reflections.)

> *"Many people who don't stutter have fears about giving a presentation or speeches and their bodies respond in the same way as people who stutter. Although for them it doesn't result in stuttering, they do sometimes repeat sounds or words, lose track of what they want to say, or have difficulty finding a specific word. They too have muscular tension throughout their body. For people who stutter, that muscle tension often finds its focus in the throat, lips, tongue, or mouth. When you are anxious you have more muscle tension and are more prone to stutter."*
>
> *"The 'fight or flight' response happens automatically and we can't extinguish it. We can, however, work to minimize it; and that can be a very useful skill in managing stuttering. An initial step is to predict when you are going to be anxious and know how your body will react. We must be attuned to our feelings and the symptoms that anxiety creates. You should reassure yourself that your anxiety is your body's natural reaction to the situation and that it is normal. This helps in learning to mitigate the fear response; after all, it is normal, but it doesn't need to take total control. If you have to answer the telephone, tell yourself that you will likely be nervous when you do and expect your brain and body to react in the usual ways. This makes the process become predictable and you will see the logic in the way you respond to the fear."*

The next step is to intercede in the process; do something differently that will help break down the habitual response pattern and make it more manageable. The client's internal dialogue might go something like, *"Oh, the phone is ringing. I am usually nervous talking on the phone and I can feel my body reacting already! Okay, that's my regular reflex when the phone rings and it has led to me stuttering in the past. But this time I'm going to take a deep breath first and begin by talking very slowly and in a relaxed manner."* The ringing phone is a trigger that becomes associated with the embarrassment of stuttering of past occasions. Left unchecked, this reflexive pattern will continue until the client does something differently. Predicting what will happen enables the client some advance time to intercede and change the outcome. This is a beginning of being able to better manage some of your fears and anxiety.

It will take practice in therapy to become proficient at managing predictable fear responses. Being able to predict them is far easier than finding yourself already in the middle of the patterned behaviors and needing to work your way out to get on top of it. But being able to work out of a block the client is already in is also a necessary skill as not all circumstances will be predictable. Understanding how your body responds to fear and anxiety makes it seem more natural, normal, and even logical. At minimum it will take "the bite" out of it.

Later, clients may benefit from identifying other nervous habits related to speaking. An effective means to approach them is to watch a video of a speech or a treatment session with the client asking him to point out features of his speaking that might lead his audience to think that he is nervous or anxious. If this task initially is too difficult for the client, watch a video of someone else and identify the indicators of anxiety that speaker displays. The process of learning to manage anxiety and stuttering also offers an opportunity to begin discussing stuttering in objective, rather than emotional terms. The client will perceive the discussion as a description of tangible, observable features of his behavior, rather than a list of "what's wrong with me."

These activities are an offshoot of the therapy theme, "Knowledge Is Power." The more you know about your stuttering, the better able you can become in overcoming it. Said differently, how can you fix something when you don't know how it works or what components aren't working properly?

Approaches to Managing Anxiety

Speech characteristics of anxiety often are observable in a client's rapid rate, abrupt voice onsets, quick or discordant breathing pattern, and forced articulation of sounds. A general approach toward countering these behaviors is for the client to speak in a slower, more disciplined, and controlled manner. For most people, speaking is relatively automatic; you have a thought and it comes out your mouth. But now, we ask the client to speak in a very disciplined, intentional way, managing his breathing, thinking about the smooth movement of the articulators, monitoring them as they come in contact with other oral structures, beginning vocalization gradually and smoothly, and, most importantly, maintaining a slow-normal, purposeful rate of speaking. The term "speaking deliberately" may characterize what is desired, and is usually quite different than "speaking automatically." Speaking becomes a much more "cerebral" process with each aspect requiring the thoughtful intention of the speaker.

Sometimes it is instructive to view and discuss the characteristics of other well-known speakers and select one for the client to emulate. *"I want you to read this aloud as if you were Mr. Rogers,"* making note of the rate, vocal softness, and ease with which he speaks. (Mr. Rogers videos are readily available on YouTube to be used as examples.) Learning is promoted by clinician modeling; show the client what you want him to do in addition to telling him. By emulating the speech of someone else, the client's attention is focused on the overall characteristics of the other person's speech pattern and not the individual components. The speech impersonation incorporates all of the character's speaking habits, not just in the single components of slow rate, gentle onset, and the like. Thus, the whole is greater than the sum of the parts.

By analogy, contrast these two approaches to teaching someone to dance the Tango for the first time. One approach would be to teach the individual movements of each foot: where to put his left foot, then his right foot, what to do with the hands, how to move the body, and where to look. This is somewhat analogous to teaching the client target use, one target at a time. A different approach would be to demonstrate the flow and sequence of dance movements used to Tango, having the dance student imitate them to the best of her ability. This is analogous to having the client impersonate another speaker's characteristics. We don't focus on the individual elements, but try to capture the general characteristics of the overall style.

The first dance instruction approach fails to teach the flow of the movements, but the second approach may perhaps not enable the student to grasp all of the subtleties of the individual moves that result in the grace and style of the dance. By analogy, the speech pathologist likely will want to incorporate both the individual components of fluent speaking and the overall flow of ongoing speech fluency in their instruction.

Another broad-based approach is to expose the client to feared speaking situations in a gradual fashion, controlling elements that position the situation as being feared. For example, in talking to a group of people, have the client stand next to you at the front of the room. Establish the fact that he will not be asked to speak, merely to stand next to you and watch the audience as you do the talking. A "safety zone" is established by comforting the client that he will not need to speak. However this still allows him to experience some of the fears associated with standing before an audience, yet he feels secure in knowing that he will not have to talk. After 10 minutes or so, speak "one-on-one" to the client in front of the group. Ask him a few questions that can be answered with "yes" or "no." Wait for him to become comfortable in this new situation. After a while, step away from his side and move toward the audience, still facing the client and continue your questioning. Ensure that the client is still relatively comfortable, then take another step back into the audience and begin asking him questions that require him to answer in longer, complete sentences. Again, after a while and ensuring that he is still comfortable, walk to the back of the room and continue the discussion with the client. In time, encourage audience members to ask questions and interact with the client. After a few minutes, bring the discussion to a conclusion and ask the client his perceptions of what had just transpired. Point out how his anxiety was dissipated by giving it time to subside; how at first, even though he was told not to speak, the anxiety was still there. But in a short time, it diminished. Note too that the speech symptoms of anxiety also diminished, and as long as he maintained a controlled manner of speaking, fluency was the usual result. Clients are usually buoyed by their success in this exercise. Even though it might be seen as a "baby step," it can be a successful experience to cling to and provide inspiration for future attempts.

Similar experiences can be devised using the telephone. Clients who are proficient using their targets in reading may be asked to read to someone unknown to them over the phone after the clinician places the call (to a prearranged person) and introduces the client and describes what he is expected to do. The client should read until he is able to use his controlled speaking for 3 to 5 minutes. The clinician concludes the call, and then reviews the performance with the client, highlighting the characteristics of his speech and the feeling of speaking without effort on the phone.

In both of these examples, the important components to emphasize are the feelings and sensations of the client while he was speaking. The clinical objective is the change the client's feelings and beliefs about speaking in front of groups or on the telephone.

Most clients measure their success by how fluent they are. The downside of that measurement is that, once disfluencies start, there is often no means of turning them around. But measuring success by focusing on managing the conditions that underlie fluency empowers the client. Fluency is a byproduct of being relaxed, and speaking in a disciplined, controlled manner. In therapy, we teach the ability to manage the conditions which effect fluency, not fluency itself.

Client Profile

Having to give a report in class almost paralyzes Jeffery with fear. He worries about it from the time he learns of the assignment and his angst seems to build from there. He often stays home on the days he is supposed to give a report. In some classes, he has agreed to do an alternative assignment so as not to have to present in class. He also lives in fear that he will be called on in class. He is a smart student, but teachers often are unaware of his capabilities. As a result, he pretty much keeps to himself and doesn't have many friends at school.

Many people who don't stutter are very anxious about giving presentations too. To worry about stuttering on top of those normal feelings only makes the situation that much more difficult. For many people, gaining confidence "performing" before an audience is a matter of having the opportunity to have repeated exposure to the situation, taking it in small, manageable steps. Jeffery might benefit from opportunities to be in front of the class for purposes other than speaking. For example, he might assist the teacher in doing classroom demonstrations, help with computer or video equipment in class, or hand out papers to classmates. These roles might gradually necessitate casual verbal responses from Jeffery, such as, "*The PowerPoint is ready*" or "*The extension cord isn't long enough.*" Approaching feared situations in gradual increments allows clients to be better at managing their anxiety in an effective way.

Overcoming Shame

Shame is the feeling engendered when someone fails to meet a society standard and is unable to do anything to change their behavior. The emotion results as much from the behavioral standard as from the feeling of not being able to change or control it. It's a feeling of helplessness and victimization. Clients sometimes feel that, "there is something wrong with me." They often avoid speaking situations because their shameful stuttering thus will be made known. It sometimes is signaled by the client's loss of eye contact when he stutters or fears he will stutter, or by lowering his head when he talks. Usually, communicative partners detect the client's disfluencies, but these body movements signal that the stuttering is wrong and in a shameful way. The client's secondary characteristics convey to the listener that something is woefully amiss and the client himself is at fault.

Making stuttering less shameful often begins with the client's belief as to the cause of his stuttering. That the cause (or causes) of stuttering is yet unknown presents both a *complexity* and an *opportunity* for the client. Earlier in this text, the client is urged to become a spokesperson and educate others about aspects of their stuttering. People suffering an ailment are usually assumed by others to be experts on the problem. Thus, the person who stutters has the opportunity to inform listeners about what is known about stuttering that points away from it being a psychological or emotional problem, and that it is not the person's fault.

Unfortunately, most who stutter are very reticent to talk about their stuttering for fear of ridicule. However, it is a somewhat ironic characteristic of human nature that, when someone is willing to acknowledge and talk about their problem, it is no longer a source of ridicule. As a point previously made, people are genuinely curious about stuttering and if it can be made a topic of intellectual discussion, it becomes the person who has done the ridiculing who is cast in a poor light, not the person who stutters. Talking about stuttering in a serious way can help to remove the shame. *"If he can talk about his stuttering in public, how bad can it be?"* Sometimes, strangers are easier to talk to than our own friends and family. Developing a script and rehearsing it with others might ease the pathway for the client to talk with friends and family about his stuttering too.

Avoidances

It is human nature to avoid situations that may lead to conflict, confrontation, or failure. Avoidance is a behavior elicited in fear; a flight response triggered by impending danger: not only a physical danger, but an emotional danger as well. Recall that fear, and the body's response to fear, creates actions that exacerbate the underlying conditions that result in stuttering. Confronted with a situation in which a client may stutter, two choices are offered: fight through it or avoid it. The client must make a conscious decision as to what he will do. Fear is a powerful emotion, so avoidance is usually chosen by default. Choosing to avoid the situation however makes the same decision even harder the next time it is encountered; it makes the fear component bigger and stronger, so the client is more likely to choose to avoid it again in the future.

To combat a pattern of avoidance, rules need to be established that effectively take away the client's choice in situations that evoke speaking fears. Making the decision in advance and establishing it as a rule increases the likelihood of confronting rather than avoiding the fear. For example, when answering the phone there is often discretion as to whether or not to say your name in answering the call. But the prospect of saying your name generates the fear of stuttering (as it has happened so many times in the past) and it is far easier to avoid it by answering the call just saying, *"Hello, Mutual Industries, how may I help you?*" However, just having to make the decision ("Should I say my name or can I get away with not saying it?") can take mental resources away from what is needed to speak in a comfortable, controlled manner to be fluent. Allowing yourself just to ask the question creates doubt, and doubt is not a friend. Establishing and living by the rigid rule ("I *ALWAYS* say my name when answering the phone.") removes the decision and removes the doubt, allowing the client to focus all of his energy into succeeding at the task at hand, "*Hello, Mutual Industries. This is Tom Smith; how can I help you?*" Asking yourself, "*Should I or shouldn't I?*" is not even part of the process—You *MUST* say your name; that's the rule. And as you must, you must then do your best to employ the targets to make it successful.

Yielding to an avoidance is usually the harder path to take in the long run. Going swimming when the water is a little cold, there are those who dive right in, and those who take little baby steps, tip-toeing progressively deeper and deeper into the chilly water while the feelings of coldness progressively climb slowly to higher parts of their body. For those who dive in, the unpleasantness lasts a matter of seconds; for the "tip-toers" who try to avoid the shock of the cold water, the pain seems to endure forever.

However, it would be difficult to advocate teaching someone to swim by throwing them into a pool. The therapeutic part of our treatment prepares the client for his encounters by ensuring that he is capable of using speech targets and moving his therapy through progressive challenges so that the targeted situation is not overwhelming. Clients should be able to be successful using appropriate speech targets, having moved through at least of few situations in which their emerging target use has been challenged. Experienced fluency clinicians appreciate that the client's developing skills will be variable and that guided practice will help them to stabilize it.

Beliefs About Stuttering

The client's experiences stuttering usually teach him many things. Beliefs develop that undermine the will and confidence of the speaker. Although these beliefs are often understandable, they need not "doom" the client's future speaking attempts as much as he allows them to. Working to dispel beliefs is often a difficult journey, but it is part of the process of regaining natural attitudes about speaking and interacting with others.

Some clients believe that they are more likely to stutter on certain sounds than others. Many avoid saying words that incorporate these feared sounds. These beliefs seriously undercut the client's confidence and ability to articulate the sounds and words fluently. When feared sounds are encountered, it is common for the speaker to react in a number of ways, such as hurrying his attempt to say the feared word/sound or using extra effort to articulate them. These natural reactions are exactly the opposite of what is required to utter them fluently. Speech is intended to be a fluid and virtually effortless motor activity. Increasing the rate of speech increases the complexity of the muscular task and coordination. Using more muscular effort distorts the dynamics of the movements, changing the coordination and movement transitions between sounds. What the client does attempting not to stutter serves to actually increase the likelihood of it occurring.

Beliefs about stuttering usually result in avoidances and fears about speaking. For those who stutter, experience can be a cruel but powerful teacher, and memories of past speaking mishaps become accentuated in memory. Beliefs, and the physical behaviors that result, often represent sizable obstacles to successful target use in therapy. Unfortunately, beliefs are usually slow to change and consequently they should be addressed as early as possible as a part of therapy.

It usually takes time for the clinician to identify and map a client's belief system. This is part of learning to talk with the patient, who is the primary source of the information.

Some Activities for Speech Goals

Activities are the heart of any treatment session and are designed to help the client make motoric changes in his speech. Speech targets are the techniques selected to address the specific characteristics of the client's stuttering. It is recommended that only one speech target be used at a time in an activity, especially in the early sessions of therapy. This helps the client better focus on a single component of his therapy and makes it easier for the clinician to monitor his performance, record data, and give feedback. Remember, it usually is important to place the exercise in a context to help the client see the application and value of the activity he is being asked to do. Some sample speech activities are offered in the section that follows.

Hot Topics

These are client monologues in response to topics prepared by the clinician.

Objective

This activity offers clients the opportunity to use their speech targets during extemporaneous speaking. Teens and adults commonly encounter situations such as this in their daily lives in which they are asked to share their opinions on a variety of topics. This activity provides practice for the client to generate speech (formulating an opinion) while using his speech targets. Over the course of therapy sessions, you can systematically require the client to speak for longer and longer periods of time.

Description

Topics written on pieces of paper by the clinician are placed in a container for client to select. Once a topic has been selected, the client must speak about it for a given amount of time (usually 2 to 3 minutes) while maintaining target use. Keep a clock or stopwatch handy so the client can be aware of the time he is required to talk. Be silent and wait for the client to continue speaking if he runs out of things to say; this will communicate to him nonverbally that he is expected to speak for a longer time. Topics should be appropriate for the individual client (adult or child) and might include ideas like:

- What would you enjoy the most about if you could be a member of the opposite sex for a whole day?
- What are your three biggest pet peeves about drivers in this town?
- Do you think listing the names and addresses of convicted criminals on the Internet is a good idea?
- Should students be allowed to use cell phones in high school?
- Should schools sell pizza and soda pop in the school cafeteria, or only healthy foods?
- If you could eat only one food for the next 6 weeks, what would you choose and why?
- Should texting while driving be outlawed?

Discussion

Clinicians might also select topics having to do with stuttering, allowing the client to discuss his feelings and beliefs about his speech while using his therapy targets. The information that is forthcoming provides the clinician with further insights into the client's perceptions and beliefs about his difficulties with stuttering. Examples might include:

- Why do people who stutter speak fluently when they sing?
- What are three things you wish everyone knew about stuttering?

Giving Directions

People are commonly asked directions by strangers needing assistance finding their way in an area that is unfamiliar to them.

In real life, the task offers several challenges inherent in being asked to provide directions. The request usually comes by surprise and from a complete stranger. Also, the client will need to think of the best route from the present location to reach the desired destination and some landmarks along the way. For many, there is the impulsive thought that the response to the request needs to made very quickly. Be sure to correct the client if he begins too quickly as that is an unproductive habit he will want to change. For this therapy activity, a local street map might be provided as a guide for the client. Because of a tendency to respond quickly, encourage the patient to take the time necessary to be accurate and use his speech targets effectively.

Objective

The client is asked to use speech targets while speaking spontaneously. Most clients find this to be a very functional activity, something that they are likely to be called on to do from time to time. The difficulty of the activity can be varied by changing the complexity of getting to a more difficult locations or needing to take detours to avoid certain obstacles, such as road closures, along the way or because of construction or travel through undesirable neighborhoods.

Description

Recruit a stranger the client does not know and prepare him or her to ask the client for directions to various sites around town. The client must provide detailed instructions to help the stranger get from the current location (Point A) to Point B using a street map or other informational resource.

Discussion

As an alternate way of utilizing this activity idea, have the client approach a stranger outside the treatment room and ask for directions to a specific landmark in the area. Have him or her ask clarifying questions about the directions to be sure they will be able to find their way, rather than just asking how to get there and saying 'thank you'. Inquire about parking and even good places to eat while they are there.

The Greeter

If you have ever shopped at Walmart you know that there is a person in a red vest who welcomes you as you enter the store. The greeter says basically the same thing over and over and over to each new person coming into the store. When called up to do something that makes you anxious, your anxiety almost always diminishes if you repeat the task many times in fairly rapid succession. But so often in life we get only one chance at doing something (like when we introduce ourselves to someone else) and there is no opportunity for the anxiety to diminish because we only say our name once (unless the person didn't understand what we said). But the greeter gets to say his welcome message over and over and over again. Over time, after numerous greetings, the client's anxiety level reduces and more natural fluency is allowed to emerge. For most who stutter, this is a unique experience.

Objective

This activity, using targets in spontaneous speech, affords the client repeated exposure to his speaking fears doing the same task over and over. For many clients, the most difficult part of speaking is getting started. At the onset, tension is the greatest and memories of past "nonsuccesses" are the sharpest. By creating the opportunity for the client to have brief, rapid, and repeated opportunities to initiate verbal interactions with others, the tension, fear, and vivid memories will diminish with successive attempts.

Description

Have the client volunteer to greet worshippers as they enter their church or at a social event. For the first few entrants, say something brief like "*hello*" or "*welcome*," using exaggerated speech targets. As time goes on, lengthen the message using the guest's name and a longer greeting message.

Discussion

Perhaps of even greater importance, be sure the client feels his nervousness and tension diminish as the time progresses. Compare the anxiety interacting with the first few people with the 50th and 100th person being greeted. For many clients, this may be the first time they have spoken and felt so at ease.

The Time Capsule

How will this era in history be remembered? People place items representative of a specific period in time into a capsule, which is buried, to be opened at a much later date. The items selected for placement in the time capsule should be the "icons" that represent what life was like during that era.

Objective

To use speech targets in extemporaneous speech. Activities frequently become more challenging when the client is required to divert mental resources (thinking about what representative items to include in the time capsule) while using targets concurrently. The client and clinician later can discuss why the client felt that each item was representative of the era.

Description

What would you put into a time capsule to help people understand what it was like to live in this period of history? The client is asked to identify 20 things he would put into the time capsule so that people 100 years from now would understand what it was like to live in this era. The items should represent those things that are of particular significance specifically to the present time. Clients sometimes have a tendency to just generate a list of items. The clinician should ask the client to explain why each item is important and what it represents about society or our culture right now. Remember, the objective is to generate speech output for the client to practice his target use. The activity necessitates that the client think and speak (using targets) at the same time.

Discussion

As an alternative, the client might be asked to select an item, song, person, or event that uniquely represents each decade over the past century. Or, he might choose 10 things to be buried with him that have been the most meaningful in his life. The challenge (or cognitive load) of this activity comes in having to generate ideas *and* use speech targets.

Pay to Play!

There frequently comes a time in therapy when it is difficult to tell if a client is truly doing the best that he is capable of doing using targets. Two approaches work toward providing temporary, stronger reinforcement to test the client's performance capabilities: one using positive reinforcers; one using quasinegative reinforcers. With children, immediate positive reinforcement can be a powerful motivator; the child earns a penny each time he uses a speech target and loses one each he doesn't use it sufficiently. At the end of the activity, he gets to take home with him all the pennies that he earned. Tokens to trade for a desirable prize will also work. This might be an ongoing contest, keeping track of his successes week by week and comparing performances.

For the adult, pennies likely won't work and most clinicians would be hard pressed to substitute 10-dollar-bills in their place! Instead, have them imagine a scenario in which they would receive a sizable electric shock each time they neglected to use a speech target or did not use it satisfactorily. In actuality, the clinician could use a small siren or bicycle horn to simulate the imagined electrical shock. The horn will help make the point be made (and the clinician won't be sued or arrested for torturing a client). In either scenario, the client's performance is likely to peak, providing insight into what the client is actually capable of doing.

Objective

This activity serves to increase target use and test the client's optimal performance ability. This is a pretty basic reinforcement strategy, but for a client who is "stuck," it can get them (and you) over the "hump."

Description

A stack of pennies (or poker chips or tokens) is placed on the table. Each time the client successfully uses a speech target to the satisfaction of the clinician, a penny is moved into the client's pile. However, one is removed each time the client neglects to use a speech target satisfactorily. The client is allowed to keep all the pennies that are left in his pile after a given period of time. Be very stringent in gauging the client's target use; "perfect is good enough!" If you can't tell that he used a target, he didn't. Chart the client's winnings each session so that he has a record to beat in addition to money to make. For many children this adds an extra level of motivation and enthusiasm.

Discussion

A discussion or summary of the findings could follow the activity. Depending on the results, the client and clinician can see whether the client needs to work harder to use targets so that, when he does, his speech will be more fluent. Alternatively, it may demonstrate that the client is working up to his capacity and perhaps another technique could be selected to develop another tool to help the client manage his fluency.

Story Sharing

The client and clinician (or other clients) rely on their imagination, taking turns telling a story that they spontaneously fabricate together.

Objective

Story sharing aims for clients to use targets during a spontaneous speaking situation. This activity encourages imagination and creativity, each of which increases the cognitive demands of the task.

Description

Participants (the clinician and clients) take turns continuing telling a story they spontaneously concoct. The clinician begins by starting the story, introducing one or two characters and the beginning of the story line. After a minute or so, the next person must continue to develop the story, building on the information already provided. Being creative (or silly) can enhance the enthusiasm for the activity. Target use is continuously the subject of the clinician's feedback and commentary.

Discussion

If the story goes too far askew or target use becomes secondary to being humorous, the clinician will need to redirect the activity. The clinician might ask one of the participants to summarize the highlights of what happened in the story or ask questions of the clients, while still maintaining target use.

Talk Show Host

Making conversation and asking questions to learn about someone new are common social activities. This activity casts one person in the role of the interviewer (or host) and one as the interviewee (or guest). The host must make conversation and learn about the guest, much like on a television talk show or at social gatherings. The interviewee may be himself, play the role of a famous person, or an individual with a special talent or having done something outrageous (like being able to walk across hot coals or having bungeed off the Empire State Building). The clinician and client take turns being the interviewer and interviewee, as both roles require different skills.

Objective

To promote target use and practice making: asking and answering questions and carrying on a conversation with someone else, while using speech targets. .

Description

The client plays the role of a talk show host and is required to ask questions of another person (the clinician or another client) to learn about aspects of their life. The person interviewed can be a real or fictional. The interviewee can play the part of someone else, like Superman, Benjamin Franklin, or anyone of their choosing. For clients who may be somewhat less verbal, it is sometimes easier for them to play the part of the interviewee, needing only to respond to questions rather than generate them. The role of the fictitious character interviewee may be defined as someone with an unusual talent (like the ability to balance a ping-pong ball on his nose while eating popcorn!). As the talk show host, the clinician questions the client about his special talent.

Discussion

Just beneath the surface, recognize that this activity parallels the conversational skills used at a social gathering or meeting new people in the workplace. Playing roles of famous or fictitious people can add an element of levity to the activity. However, most clients both enjoy and see the utility in this activity.

How Does That Work?

People often are asked to explain something that they are knowledgeable of or know something about that others do not. In this activity, the client is asked to describe the process by which something works or how it is made. It could be as simple as making coffee or as complicated as explaining how an air conditioner works; or even having the client fabricate an explanation for something he really does not understand.

Objective

This activity can be modified to increase the cognitive load for clients. It requires them to provide information or instruction in a logical way while using speech targets at the same time. The topic can be adjusted to the specific expertise or interests of the client, from making toast, providing instructions to make a paper airplane, or explaining how an airplane is able to fly.

Another level of complexity can be added by having the client do something physical at the same time, such as walking at a very quick pace. Respiration patterns for physical exertion can conflict with breathing patterns for speech. Exercise requires more rapid inspiration/expiration cycles. For speech, the exhalation phase of the breathing cycle is much longer than the inhalation phase. As a consequence, speaking while engaged in a form of physically activity places the speaker in the position of needing to accommodate the needs for breathing and speaking simultaneously.

Description

The client is asked to instruct the clinician how to make something. The selection of the "something" to be explained enables the clinician to vary the level of difficulty of the task.

To tap other modalities, the clinician can describe how to do something first and then require the client to explain it back; this may be beneficial with clients who tend not to talk much. Searching the Internet, picture instructions (instructions without words) can be found which can serve to guide a client who is not particularly talkative. The client's task then becomes explaining what the character in the illustrations is doing. To find them, type "wordless workshop" into an Internet search engine to locate pictorial instructions.

To add difficulty to this task, interrupt the client frequently while he is explaining something a little complicated, like how a compact fluorescent light bulb works and why you can't use a dimmer switch with one; or challenge the facts he presents as he discusses the topic. The clinician can interrupt the client using a quick rate of speech to try to distract him from using his targets.

Discussion

Clients frequently lose focus on the most important aspect of this activity, that of using speech targets. Keep the client working diligently on managing his speech. The best way to do that is by giving a lot of feedback. Sometimes, an auditory signal or gesture can be used as a reminder to use targets more appropriately. As a rule of thumb, if it's not perfect, let the client know right away and have him do it again correctly. Practicing the targets incorrectly makes little sense and will not be productive. Some clients become more interested in giving the instructions than using their targets. Don't let that happen; it can get out of hand easily and then you're not doing your job.

Reading Famous Speeches

It sometimes is beneficial for the client to "lose himself" in a part or role he is playing. In fact, some renowned actors, such as James Earl Jones, stutter in real life, but much less so when acting a role.

Objective

Find the text to a famous speech, like Martin Luther King's "I Have a Dream" Speech or Lincoln's "Gettysburg Address." For many clients, reading aloud is an easier mode of speaking and they do so more fluently. Rather than just reading, the client is asked to "become the person" who delivered the speech, in other words, read the speech as if he were King or Lincoln. To get "in character" may require the client to change his regular speaking pattern." This presents an opportunity to speak as someone else and act out the part. Becoming someone else can temporarily free the client from his psychological baggage and his self-imposed limitations. This takes advantage of one of the phenomena of stuttering; that people who stutter may not stutter when acting or playing the role of someone other than themselves.

Description

Using speech targets, the client reads lines from a famous speech, trying to emulate the person who actually gave the speech. Generally, the more he "lets go" and becomes the other person, the less he will stutter.

Use caution that the client does not start to use "other voices" in his own speech! The intent of this activity is to enable the client to explore fluency, not to change his personality or use tricks to be fluent.

Discussion

For many who stutter, playing a role or speaking with an accent significantly enhances their fluency. However, this is not the intended outcome of therapy; we want only to "borrow it" to enhance the client's fluency, change his perspective on stuttering, and build his confidence as a speaker. Some clients attempt to speak in a different way (with an accent, a different voice quality, or with a different pattern of intonation and inflections); this is neither an intended nor a desirable outcome. In the end, the client needs to be himself and able to manage his own fluency.

Changing Places

Having the client become the clinician and the clinician become the client can be fun and informative as the (real) clinician can gain insights into the ways the (real) client perceives his therapy. The client has amassed a good deal of experience in therapy over the many sessions he has already attended and is familiar with being on the "receiving end" or playing the learner's role in therapeutic interactions. But now, when faced with the responsibility of guiding and teaching "a client," he will likely gain additional insight into his responsibility to better manage his own stuttering, but also helping the clinician to stutter smarter (use targets better).

Objective

This activity is designed to increase the client's awareness of his disfluencies and improve self-monitoring skills. This is accomplished by switching roles in therapy, where the client becomes the clinician and the clinician poses as the client, intentionally emulating the client's therapy behaviors, such as insufficiently or inaccurately using speech targets during activities.

Description

The client and clinician trade roles in therapy; the clinician becomes the client and is required to use speech targets during typical therapeutic activities. The client must identify and describe the disfluencies evidenced by the clinician and/or instances when fluency targets were used (or should have been used). The clinician emulates the target use errors commonly made by the client while she reads or speaks. The clinician does not need to stutter in the same way as the client as some clients may feel they are being mimicked. But the clinician should neglect to use targets periodically, or use them incorrectly, and should offer the same explanations (excuses) for not using targets as the client might normally do.

Discussion

Children usually like becoming the teacher and being in charge of the session. Many, however, find it hard to stay on task and perhaps build a better appreciation for your job as the therapist. Conversely, it can help the clinician appreciate the encumbrance and challenge that using targets presents to clients as they try to communicate!

Don't Say It! That Word's Taboo!

This activity is designed to add an element of mental challenge to speaking. As speaking is almost automatic most of the time, an additional element of difficulty is added by specifying parameters of words that cannot be used in utterances. The consequence is that a good deal more effort selecting words must go into the planning process during a conversation. This has the impact of slowing the rate of speaking as added time is needed to think of appropriate synonyms for the "taboo" words. The word search can take resources away from target use; thus the client has the competing needs of making frequent changes in sentence formulation and remembering to use speech targets when appropriate.

Objective

This speaking task increases the cognitive load, adding complexity to test the client's ability to use the speech targets. It can be practiced in conversation, extemporaneous speaking, or reading. It focuses on making speaking a very controlled, rather than automatic, act.

Description

The client is "forbidden" to say specific words in conversation or monologues. The clinician specifies the parameters of the taboo words, perhaps words starting with the letter "s," for example, or a word that will be critical and heavily used in the upcoming conversation. The client must maintain a conversation with the clinician or describe something without using the forbidden words. The activity can be made harder by specifying that words with "s" in it, in any position, cannot be used. In general, broadening the taboo criteria makes the task harder, like not starting a sentence with a word beginning with a vowel.

This activity makes speaking harder in that the client needs to think about managing their stuttering *and* scan ahead for forbidden words. It also serves to greatly slow the process of speaking, which is another theme in therapy. The idea of making speaking a more "thoughtful" process is promoted.

Discussion

There are innumerable twists to this activity, such as starting each consecutive sentence with the next consecutive letter of the alphabet; so the first sentence would start with a word beginning the letter "a"; the second sentence would start with the letter "b," and so on. Remember that the object is to challenge the client's ability to use speech targets during the conversation.

Introductions

Introducing yourself and your friends to others is a common occurrence in our social and business lives. For most who stutter, saying their name can be a challenge under the pressures of making introductions with strangers. Even introducing other people to one another can be daunting. For most, a history of difficult past experiences haunts them and their fears of stuttering and anxieties begin even before they utter their first word. Attempts at speaking reflect this anxiety as the client rushes his rate and forces out feared words.

Objective

This activity helps clients manage their speech targets in common social situations. It is very common for people who stutter to let their fears overwhelm their discipline speaking when making introductions, particularly introducing themselves. This exercise can provide multiple opportunities for the client to learn that he can speak in a relaxed, disciplined manner in a situation that he typically finds to be stressful.

Description

Have the client introduce himself to others using speech targets. Because most clients have had a strong history of difficulty with introductions, it may be prudent to work with the client on some socially appropriate strategies to construct a new approach to this task. Because of their fears, many clients approach the task with speed and muscular force in getting their name out. To manage the situation differently, you may instruct the client to let the other person say their name first. This breaks up the habit pattern and gives the client more time to relax himself. Instead of starting his introduction by immediately saying his name, the client might begin by saying something like, "*Hi Tammy, it's so very nice to meet you. My name is Michael and I work in the accounting department.*" The added time is used to enlist a more disciplined approach to speaking by breaking up the habitual pattern of reacting to the situation in a different, but socially acceptable way.

As an alternative to this activity, have the client spend a few minutes learning about someone else by asking questions of them. For clients who might be a little socially awkward or inexperienced, it's sometimes helpful to provide a structured format for this portion of the activity, giving the client a list of specific questions to ask. Then have the client introduce the person he just interviewed to you, as if he were introducing a friend to you, stating the person's name and a few of the things he learned about them from talking with them a few moments before.

Discussion

Even though it may appear unusual, have your client introduce himself to the same person three or four times consecutively. For most, doing the same task repeatedly, one after another, usually sees the client's tension level fall. Draw attention to the decrease in tension and to the feel of speaking (saying his own name) in an easy, relaxed manner.

If it is feasible, audio- or video-record the interactions so that the client can review his performance with you. This will enable him to see how his anxiety impacts his stuttering and the little signs of tension that may be communicated nonverbally.

Most clients find this to be a very functional activity as it is something they are likely to be called on to do on their job or at social events. The three most important components involved in this activity are: (1) breaking up the old habit pattern, (2) speaking in a very slow, relaxed manner, and (3) demonstrating speaking as a volitional activity rather than a reflex.

Some Activities for Emotive Goals

A wide range of emotional issues in stuttering should be addressed in therapy. They include the client's attitudes about speaking and stuttering, concern about the perceptions of others, guilt and shame of what the client's stuttering may represent to others, dealing with the fears and anxieties about speaking, overcoming the past negative experiences stuttering, and worry and despair about the future. Both specific and global issues need to be addressed. Some clinicians do not feel comfortable dealing with these issues, but they are of critical importance to the end product and outcome of therapy. Unless they are adequately addressed, it is likely that the client will relapse and his stuttering will return. None of the following activities will, by itself, enable to client to "fix" what is "broken." Instead, each of the following activities may be used as an avenue to begin a discussion, enabling the clinician to counsel the client and address the issues most pertinent in his stuttering.

One avenue toward dispelling the myths and misinformation about stuttering is to build the client's knowledge base about stuttering. Often, the feelings of shame and guilt are reflections of inaccurate information about stuttering, such as stuttering being an outward manifestation of a deep-seated emotional problem. Part of the approach in addressing this issue is helping the client to become an educator who is able to teach others about stuttering. The following activities give the clinician an opportunity to educate the client to become an educator himself.

Write a Booklet About Stuttering

This activity can help the client organize and script his thoughts about stuttering. It also can serve as an avenue for the clinician to educate the client about stuttering, reaffirming his accurate knowledge and reorienting any misconceptions or misinformation. Being able to discuss stuttering as an intellectual topic often enables the client to defuse unpleasant situations by educating those with whom he interacts. Clients' knowledge of stuttering often contains inaccuracies and misinformation. The ability to discuss stuttering begins with a good foundation of information.

Objective

Begin educating the client by discussing the aspects of stuttering that are important for people to know. A first step may be to establish an outline or table of contents for the booklet on stuttering. This serves to organize the client's thoughts about stuttering and establish a structure of information to talk to others about it. This exercise also enables the clinician to assess the client's current understanding of his stuttering and then supplement his knowledge or correct misinformation.

Description

Explain the purposes of writing the booklet about stuttering; for example, to become expert on stuttering, to be better able to talk with others about stuttering, or to help others better understand what stuttering is and how it affects people. Encourage the client by letting him know when listeners get beyond the "surprise" of finding out that he stutters that there is actually a good deal of honest curiosity about it. People are interested in learning more and are intrigued by many of the curiosities about stuttering, such as that people who stutter don't stutter when they sing and when they are alone. Engaging others intellectually about stuttering elevates the interaction beyond it being the subject of ridicule to a topic of intellectual curiosity.

Begin by developing a list of the things that the client feels are important for others to know about stuttering. Next, organize the list into categories (like, different types of disfluencies, difficult situations such as talking on the phone, challenging situations such as introducing yourself, etc). Then, organize the categories into chapters of the booklet and develop a table of contents.

Discussion

This activity can help identify things the client doesn't know about his stuttering (like what causes stuttering or that it has a genetic basis for some people) and can become the impetus to "fill in" these missing pieces of information. Writing the booklet is usually a long-term project that develops with the client's understanding of his stuttering. Working on parts of the book also can be a meaningful homework assignment, requiring the client to do more reading and research on aspects of stuttering so that he will be more knowledgeable. For younger clients, the information and explanations can be geared to their level. Remember, the objective is to enable the client to discuss his stuttering as an intellectual topic with others. Many children who stutter have given an informational presentation about their stuttering to their classmates.

Scripting a Cause of Stuttering

The cause of stuttering is often a kernel issue for those who stutter. Relating to the previous activity, having the opportunity to gather factual information and be able to articulate a well-reasoned explanation of this disorder can carry a good deal of weight toward combating the ridicule of others and forming a sound explanation of stuttering for the client himself.

Objective

Many who stutter are sensitive to characterizations of stuttering as being a mental disorder or something that the person who stutters does intentionally. Thus, the cause of stuttering itself can be a major issue. Not knowing the precise cause of stuttering (which is presently the case) can keep inaccuracies about stuttering (like it being an emotional problem or caused by nervousness) alive. But, despite not knowing the cause, a well-constructed statement about what is known about stuttering, and what is known *not* to be factual, does provide a defense against arguments constructed on misperceptions and information proven to be untrue.

It is not common to find people to be joyous to learn that a condition they manifest has been discovered to have a genetic origin. But such was the case for many who stutter when research found that there was a genetic abnormality in the subject population of people who stutter that was researched. The joy found in this news stemmed from the adjudication that their stuttering was not a symptom of a psychological problem, a mental disorder, or something the person who stutters did intentionally; it's genetic!

When the person who stutters becomes a source of knowledge for others, he elevates his position and lessens the perceptions of pity and ridicule. Deservedly so or not, society attributes an inherent sense that a person with a malady is knowledgeable and informed about the disorder he has, he is an expert. But being ridiculed and having nothing to say in rebuttal is a painfully weak position. Developing a script for the client regarding the cause of stuttering is empowering and transforms him to become an educator and the provider of information about stuttering.

Description

Imagine you have a condition that society sees as "different" and undesirable and it feels like there is nothing that you can do to change it. The condition is not immediately obvious to others until you speak; there are no visible signs of your difference, except sometimes when you talk. Most people would try their best to conceal this difference because they feel ashamed that something is wrong with them and they cannot do anything to fix it. This attitude is conveyed to each person you come into contact with; you are a helpless victim of the disorder.

Developing a script enables the client to have his information in readily accessible form. Having the client write it helps to organize his thoughts. Rehearsing it helps for the thoughts and ideas to flow more easily when the opportunity arises to share it with others.

Discussion

In many instances the client not only doesn't want to talk about his stuttering, he doesn't know what to say. Constructing a script helps clients understand their stuttering, and particularly its cause. Armed with a script, the client can begin to say something about their problem; they become a dispenser of knowledge, rather than a victim of ignorance.

To the surprise of many a person who stutters, their listener becomes interested in knowing more about the topic of stuttering and any feelings of ridicule the client anticipates vanish and the shame dissolves.

Parallel Feelings

Sometimes, our empathy for the feelings of others is a catalyst that brings out our own feelings. Watching someone else with a disability, we project how we might feel and deal with such an adversity. The concerns which we might express reveal our inner feelings, perceptions, and sometimes misconceptions. This happens when one person who stutters watches another. The feelings and emotions that come to mind in empathy for the other person are usually reflective of the person's own feelings about their situation.

Objective

Many clients find it very difficult to talk about how they feel about their stuttering. In some cases, they may have not allowed themselves to think about it because it is painful and just easier "not to go there." As a consequence, many who stutter may not be able to express their feelings about their stuttering. For others, it may be hard to put their feelings into words. Involvement in group therapy or support groups can be an effective means of exploring and developing feelings about stuttering among participants. By listening to other group members, they learn how their peers who stutter feel about their stuttering. In some cases, they find that others have feelings similar to theirs, whereas others likely feel quite differently. For those who have not revealed their feelings, the group discussion can be a safe place to do so. For those who are yet to discover their feelings, they can begin to formulate ideas by acknowledging the similarities and differences between their own feelings and the feelings others have expressed.

Where groups are not available, clients can compare their feelings to others by watching videos of people who stutter and discussing what they observed with the clinician. The client might be asked how he thinks the person on the video feels in the situation and to explain why he thinks the person feels that way. It seems to be human nature to find it easier to talk about someone else and his problems than to talk about ourselves and our problems; this is especially true with stuttering. But, either way, the objective is to increase awareness and be better able to articulate the feelings and emotions about stuttering.

Description

After viewing a video/DVD of someone who stutters, the client describes how the character who stuttered in a video felt in the situation portrayed. The comments made by the client usually reflect his experience with his own stuttering as much or more than the character in the video. Thus, the client is actually talking about his own stuttering and his own feelings about it.

Discussion

Care needs to be taken watching videos of other clients who stutter that patient confidentiality is not violated. Getting a client's written permission is advisable. However, many videos of people who stutter available on Internet sources such as YouTube. Other commercially available videos include, "Voices in Exile" or "Transcending Stuttering: The Inside Story." These sources safeguard the clinician by avoiding potential patient confidentiality risks.

Watching videos of others is often a beneficial starting point because it seems to always be easier to talk about others than reveal things about ourselves. However, the client's comments about the person in the video usually reflect his own, therefore, are often quite revealing. The challenge usually comes in getting the client started talking; afterward his thoughts often flow more easily.

Drawing a Picture of the Stutter

Many mediums of expression allow clients who stutter to express their feelings; one of them is through artwork. It is not their artistic ability that is of concern as much as providing a vehicle of expression. Whether a full color rendering or a stick man, having a means and a reason to discover and describe the client's feelings is the clinician's therapeutic concern.

Objective

The aim of this activity is to develop the client's ability to access and express his feelings about his stuttering. Drawing a picture of stuttering enables the client to depict aspects of stuttering that he will then explain. The picture is considered a starting point for a deeper discussion of the client's perspectives and experiences with his disfluent speech and his feelings about stuttering. The information that stems from this activity can help the clinician understand the client's situation and identify needs to be addressed in future sessions.

Description

The client is given a piece of paper and a pencil (or other drawing instrument) and asked to draw a picture of his stutter in 3 to 4 minutes. After completion, the client is asked to talk about what the picture represents.

Discussion

For some clients, drawing is a medium that makes it easier for them to discuss their perceptions; whether the picture serves as a distraction or somehow validates their opinions is not always clear. What is clear is that new information is usually forthcoming. Clients do not seem reluctant to explain their drawings. Clinicians should remember that the client's perceptions are the reality he perceives; accurate or inaccurate, that is the world in which he lives.

Video Self-Assessment

For most people, watching themselves on video can be difficult. Sometimes we are our own toughest critic and seeing the reality as others see us can be rather confrontational, even upsetting, for many. Critically watching yourself on video can also be very motivating. Seeing yourself and not liking what you see can be the catalyst for a very rapid behavior change.

Objective

Having the client view himself on video can provide the opportunity for him to see his stuttering as others do. The goal of this activity is to improve the client's self-awareness and ability to look at the characteristics of his stuttering objectively. This knowledge is power.

Description

Video record the client speaking for 5 to 10 minutes using a small (pocket) video camera. Then, the client and clinician can review the video together. The image from most pocket video cameras can be enlarged by viewing them on a laptop or desktop computer. The video could also be downloaded and given to the client to review for homework.

Discussion

Watching a video can be quite confrontation for clients who stutter, seeing themselves for perhaps the first time as others see them. Some who stutter protect themselves by "turning a blind eye to" (purposefully ignoring) their stuttering as if it didn't happen. This self-defense mechanism shields their ego from the truth that all others see, but it spares the client from dealing with the realities of his own stuttering. For these clients, seeing themselves on video shatters their "reality" and they find watching the truth on video to be very disturbing. You likely will note this if the client has difficulty watching the video. In this case, the clinician might alter the activity by muting the sound on the video and asking the client to identify instances when he stuttered and what the behaviors were that marked his instances of disfluency. The lesson then becomes one of working toward minimizing the outward, secondary characteristics of stuttering to make the client's disfluencies less noticeable.

Clients sometimes are overly critical of aspects of their speaking behaviors that are not really germane to their stuttering. To prevent this, provide the client with specific things to look for while reviewing his video performance, such as tension in the lips, eye contact, his rate of speech, or other characteristics specific to his stuttering. This can help focus attention on desired behaviors and directing the client's learning so that he can see exactly what you are seeing.

Give the client the chance to critique his performance first (before the clinician makes any comments); this will afford a degree of "self-protection" in the process. It can take clients three or more times watching their video before they are able to focus on the important, salient features of their stuttering. Many clients find this very confrontational; for the first time, they see just what everyone else sees. You'll note that some will have a great deal of difficulty watching their video, often casting their eyes in another direction, almost in disgust or shame. However, for others, this can be a significant source of motivation. Watching yourself give a speech or giving a presentation you will likely notice "little things" about your performance that can be upsetting; things like saying "*okay*" too often or playing with your hair while you are speaking, or rocking back and forth. But watching yourself a second and third time allows you to see other things (content issues) that are likely more important. Giving the client specific behaviors to observe and evaluate from the beginning likely will expedite the process.

The Fluency Fantasy

Some clients lose hope that their stuttering might someday improve, enabling them to do more with their life. Others have given up the dream of being able to communicate effectively or being able to accomplish things that they once had wanted. This activity can help them restore the vision of what they may someday become or begin to construct some new goals. It can be a useful tool in re-energizing a client who has been in therapy for a while.

Objective

The aim of this activity is to develop a vision of what the client's life would be like if he no longer stuttered. Sometimes people give up on their dreams because an obstacle seems too difficult to overcome. The purpose of this activity is twofold: to begin constructing a realistic dream for the future and to recognize that the only obstacle to attaining that dream might be the client himself.

Description

The question is posed to the client, "What would your life be like if you no longer stuttered? What would you do differently? How would this change your current life plan?" A discussion of the client's response can guide him to recognize that no one else is telling them he cannot do something, but that it's coming from within. This may provide an opportunity to develop a goal that is meaningful to the client that can be worked toward collaboratively with the clinician.

Sometimes, a goal needs to be broken down into smaller, more manageable steps. Using stories of others with a handicap or disability who have succeeded in spite of obstacles as examples can provide additional motivation. Helping the client to step outside of his comfort zone is the quickest way for him to grow.

Discussion

Many clients pay homage at the altar of the "fluency god." They feel that their imperfection, stuttering, is holding them from doing many things they would like to accomplish in their lives. From their perspective, in order to be successful, their speech needs to be fluent before they are willing to venture forward. Even if the content of what they say isn't witty or lacks meaningful information, they equate the fluency of their speech with being successful and deem it to be the most important attribute in verbal interactions.

It also takes courage to acknowledge that others are not the obstacles holding you back from your dream. For others at the end of therapy who can capably manage their fluency, their stuttering no longer serves as the reason or excuse why they have not yet accomplished the things in life that are important to them—why they haven't volunteered to be their daughter's softball coach or chaired a committee at work. For some, becoming fluent is a scary prospect as there is no longer a reason not to do the things they have been stymied from doing in the past. There is no longer the "stuttering excuse" to fall back on. You would think this would be a happy problem, but clients may need added support or counseling to move forward in their lives as fluent speakers.

Most Embarrassing Moments

Being able to laugh at yourself or your stuttering demonstrates a certain level of self-confidence and self-assuredness. Learning not to take stuttering jokes personally requires building a tougher skin. But being able to see the humor in things that involve stuttering may be an important issue for therapy. When the client and clinician share stories of times when they were embarrassed (the client about his stuttering and the clinician about their various life predicaments), the stage is set to be able to see beyond one's own narrow perspective.

Objective

The purpose of this activity is to desensitize the client to his stuttering and begin to develop a sense of objectivity about it. Being able to take the perspective of others and see humor in situations that involve stuttering is a big step for most who stutter. It requires the client to be able to pull back some of the personal feelings attached to his stuttering and the stuttering of others.

Description

Begin by having the client draw a picture depicting an embarrassing stuttering moment he has experienced. The clinician may sketch one of her personally embarrassing moment too to show that everyone gets themselves into difficult situations and the ability to laugh at yourself (at least a little) is part of how people learn to cope.

Holding up the picture, (artistic talent not required) the artist tells the story of the incident in greater detail, describes how he felt, and what he learned that might help the next time. As the clinician, you can use this opportunity to problem-solve with the client in case something similar happens again. Being able to have an open discussion about stuttering and explore feelings is a part of the therapeutic process.

Discussion

With some clients it's important that they know that others get embarrassed too when things in life go wrong and that they are able to laugh at the situation and themselves. This activity also works well in groups, as everyone gets in the spirit of sharing and learning how others feel and cope with their "humanness."

> *A young man who stuttered decided to take parachute lessons. In the plane with his parachute strapped on, the instructor gave the young man the command to, "Count to 10 and pull the cord to open the parachute." He pushed the young student out of the airplane door. The instructor could hear his student on the way down counting . . . "On-on-on-on-on-on-**one**, t-t-t-t-t-t-t-t-t-t-t-t-tw-tw-tw-two-two-**two**, th-th-th-th-th-th-thr-thr-thr-**three**, . . . "*

Life Line

It's important for clinicians to understand a client's experiences stuttering and how stuttering has impacted his life. This activity provides the opportunity for the client to tell her about selected segments of his life and the ways his stuttering has impacted it.

Objective

The activity provides the structure for the client to recall various points in his life and talk about his stuttering at that moment in time. Being able to discuss these occasions is likely to be more important than using speech targets, so focus on the content in Life Line, and save work on target use for speech target activities.

Description

The client is provided with a piece of paper with a time line drawn across the sheet (Figure 4–1). Five or six discrete periods of time are indicated on the paper and the client is asked to talk about what his life and his stuttering were like at that specific time. The sample provided identifies six points on the timeline representing the following events:

- A major world event that took place around the time of your birth
- Something that happened when you started school
- Something that happened in high school related to your speech
- Your first real job (the interview, how you felt, etc.)
- What you are doing right now, this past week?
- What you will be doing 5 years from now (how will your life be different) as your stuttering improves?

This activity lends itself well to groups in which each group member can explain their story to the rest of the group. Members thus compare the differences and similarities of their own situation.

Discussion

For many who stutter, it is important to be able to tell others of their experiences and their suffering with stuttering; it's part of the therapy. The clinician should remember that the facts of client's story are not to be challenged. It is the client's reality. It also is not the clinician's job to fix what has happened in the past. Therapy may work toward different ways of interpreting past events at some point in the future, but it is usually a mistake to try to do that initially. Attempts to do so can easily be interpreted as the clinician not

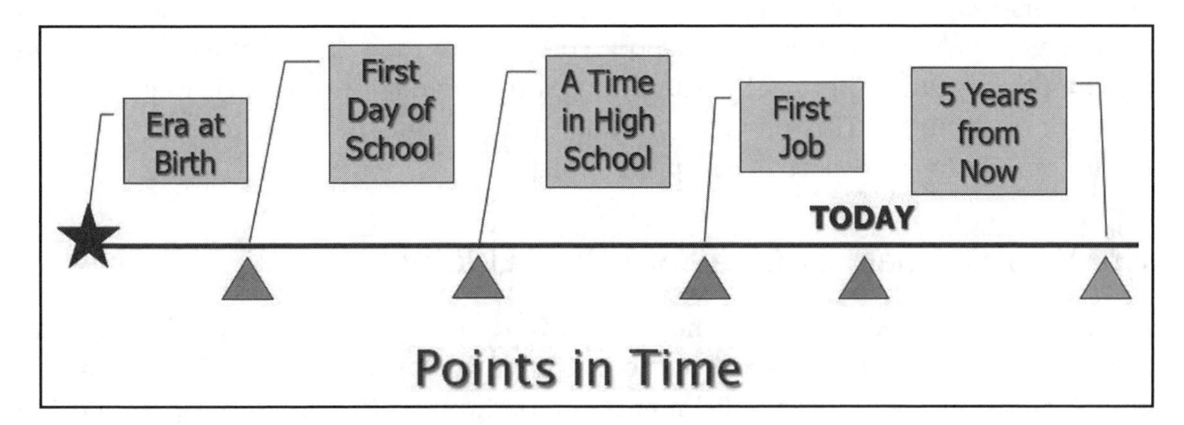

Figure 4–1. Life line activity.

understanding the client or being unwilling to accept that what he is saying to be true; as a result, the client will likely stop telling his story. Take the process one step at a time. The first step is the telling of the story; encourage the client to talk and explain his perceptions of events as completely as possible.

Reading Emotive Writings

Many people who stutter have written about their feelings and experiences stuttering. Reading these essays can stimulate and develop a client's thinking about his own stuttering; some may be similar to the author's, whereas others likely differ. But, either way, the client reflects about his feelings by comparing them with the feelings of others.

Objective

Similar to group therapy or watching a video of someone else who stutters, reading is another medium through which a client can connect with his feelings about his stuttering.

Description

Have the client read the writings of others who stutter. Some clients can use speech targets when reading aloud. For others, using speech targets may interfere with their comprehension of the passage or the ability to think about what they are reading. Ask the client to summarize the writer's viewpoint or experiences after he completes reading it. Then determine in what ways he shares the author's perspectives or has had experiences similar to what he has read about. The client's responses can be the basis of future discussions about his feelings.

Discussion

This activity also works well as a homework assignment: reading two or three essays, then writing about the similarities and differences between the client's viewpoint and the authors' perspectives. Essays can be found on the Internet at sites such as the Stuttering Homepage (http//:www.stutteringhomepage.com). Encourage the client to write his own essay about a certain aspect of his stuttering. Some clients journal each week for their homework assignment. This provides valuable insights for the clinician and helps the client become more introspective about his speech.

Write Your Obituary or Give Your Own Eulogy

This activity is intended to provide the client with an opportunity to assess his life (thus far) and become motivated to change the course of his future. The activity requires the client to communicate his accomplishments and perhaps realize that there is a good deal of time left to accomplish things that he feels are important and as yet incomplete.

Objective

This enables the client to take stock of his life and put stuttering into a broader perspective. Although this activity seems somewhat morbid on the surface, it is intended to be "spun" by the clinician into a vehicle to motivate the client's future efforts toward overcoming his stuttering in the process.

Description

The client is instructed to write his own eulogy or obituary, detailing the accomplishments for which he will be remembered. It is important to include a statement about how his stuttering "wound up" affecting his life, whether or not he let stuttering interfere with his life's goals, ambitions, and accomplishments. This can help the client to determine how much of his life he is willing to forgo because of his stuttering and how much he is willing to battle it in order to succeed.

Discussion

This activity serves as a basis for further discussion as well as setting goals and re-enlisting motivation. For some clients, it will highlight the degree to which stuttering has held them back and what they have sacrificed as a result of stuttering. It is the clinician's responsibility to make "lemonade" from these "lemons" by encouraging the client to fight to accomplish what he can, in spite of his stuttering.

Summary

Activities provide the client the chance to improve his use of targets in a controlled environmental speaking context and opportunities to change his feelings, attitudes, and beliefs about stuttering—addressing the two sides to the problem of stuttering. The client needs the clinician's feedback and advice to guide him in both areas. Clients who have been successful in stuttering therapy report that, regardless of the approach used, the most important component of their therapy was their clinician. The activities you design and use in therapy will reflect your philosophy of therapy. Be prepared to discuss the importance of each step of your work with the client so he knows and understands what he is doing. Your attitudes, motivation, and support will make the difference.

Index

A

C